Feeling Sick

Contemporary Hispanic and Lusophone Cultures

This series aims to provide a forum for new research on modern and contemporary hispanic and lusophone cultures and writing. The volumes published in Contemporary Hispanic and Lusophone Cultures reflect a wide variety of critical practices and theoretical approaches, in harmony with the intellectual, cultural and social developments that have taken place over the past few decades. All manifestations of contemporary hispanic and lusophone culture and expression are considered, including literature, cinema, popular culture, theory. The volumes in the series will participate in the wider debate on key aspects of contemporary culture.

12 H. Rosi Song, *Lost in Transition: Constructing Memory in Contemporary Spain*

13 Andrés Zamora, *Featuring Post-National Spain: Film Essays*

14 Paul Julian Smith, *Dramatized Societies: Quality Television in Spain and Mexico*

15 Joan Ramon Resina, *The Ghost in the Constitution: Historical Memory and Denial in Spanish Society*

16 José Colmeiro, *Peripheral Visions/Global Sounds: From Galicia to the World*

17 Regina Galasso, *Translating New York: The City's Languages in Iberian Literatures*

18 Daniel F. Silva, *Anti-Empire: Decolonial Interventions in Lusophone Literatures*

19 Luis I. Prádanos, *Postgrowth Imaginaries: New Ecologies and Counterhegemonic Culture in Post-2008 Spain*

20 Liz Harvey-Kattou, *Contested Identities in Costa Rica: Constructions of the* Tico *in Literature and Film*

21 Cecilia Enjuto-Rangel, Sebastiaan Faber, Pedro García-Caro, and Robert Patrick Newcomb, eds, *Transatlantic Studies: Latin America, Iberia, and Africa*

22 Ana Paula Ferreira, *Women Writing Portuguese Colonialism in Africa*

23 Esther Gimeno Ugalde, Marta Pacheco Pinto and Ângela Fernandes, eds, *Iberian and Translation Studies: Literary Contact Zones*

24 Ben Bollig, *Moving Voices: Poetry on Screen in Argentine Cinema*

25 Daniel F. Silva, *Empire Found: Racial Identities and Coloniality in Twenty-First-Century Portuguese Popular Cultures*

Feeling Sick

The Early Years of AIDS in Spain

DEAN ALLBRITTON

LIVERPOOL UNIVERSITY PRESS

First published 2023 by
Liverpool University Press
4 Cambridge Street
Liverpool
L69 7ZU

British Library Cataloguing-in-Publication data
A British Library CIP record is available

ISBN 978-1-80207-804-6 cased

Typeset in Borges by
Carnegie Book Production, Lancaster
Printed and bound by CPI Group (UK) Ltd, Croydon CR0 4YY

Contents

Acknowledgments

As I suspect holds true for many academic projects, this book began as a way to process something about myself. As a queer adolescent growing up in South Georgia, the specter of HIV/AIDS always loomed large; as I grew older, regardless of the truth of the matter, illness felt like an inevitability, magnetized by my sexuality. AIDS was a damning lodestar. Part of this book has been an exercise in understanding this fear as well as the politics, people, and institutions that have helped foment and sustain it.

I have been fortunate to have been supported at every step in this process by a wide net of family, friends, colleagues, and institutions. At Colby College, the Center for the Arts and Humanities and the Humanities Division funded course development grants and travel to Spain to hunt down archival materials. My colleagues across campus but particularly in Cinema Studies, Spanish, and Women's, Gender, and Sexuality Studies have listened to talks and offered valuable insight to this project. My students have given their best thinking through HIV/AIDS, particularly the classes 'Queer Spain' (Spring 2018 and Spring 2020) and 'Medical Spanish' (Fall 2020 and Fall 2022). My research assistants through the years (who continually and curiously ask when the book is coming out) can now breathe easier knowing that their work was not in vain: Oscar Mancinas, Bob Bernhart, Alexander Morris, Spencer Jeffrey, and James Burnett. May it forever be known that Luke Bowe transcribed the entirety of Jess Franco's script, including every error and misspelling.

I have presented this work over many years now, and each time have learned more about the project. I am particularly thankful to the panels and audiences at annual conferences of the Society for Cinema and Media Studies, Visible Evidence, the European Network for Cinema Studies, and the Society for Literature, Science, and the Arts. I am grateful to Sarah Thomas for inviting me to give a lecture on hemophilia at Brown University, and to Luke Bowe for his generous invitation to think alongside Lina Meruane and Miguel Caballero at New York University.

I began this project as an archival neophyte, and soon found a haven and warm reception with Victor León, the head archivist of *Documentación* at the SIDA STUDI archives. This book would be woefully incomplete without his careful help, rapid response, and immense knowledge. The special collections librarians of San Francisco State University were both patient and kind as I pored through their documents, offering sympathy and understanding when the materials were too overwhelming. Yolanda Martínez Villamar at Radiotelevisión Española was a boon in revealing the untold and undigitized treasures in the RTVE archives. I cannot thank these archival sources enough for holding on to our past.

A book project like this one is made of people. Alejandro Melero has read more of my work than anyone else, and never ceases to champion my attempts at articulating something about the cultures of Spain. His imprint is all over this book. Tom Whittaker, frequent collaborator and friend, listened to years of this work and read selections from it. Jon Snyder helped me process the intricacies of queer care in the 1980s. Theodore Kerr continuously shows me how this type of work can and must be done, and the social imperatives that accompany it. Both Sarah Thomas and Mary Kate have cheered me on and listened to every doubt with patience, and often provided wisdom and laughs just between us girls. Julián Daniel Gutiérrez once asked one of the most difficult questions about my work, and that question has subsequently helped me understand my articulation of the history of AIDS. I'm so thankful to him for sharing his micro-histories with me. Miguel Caballero has taught me much about illness, AIDS, and authenticity. Chris Walker knew little of the book but was an earnest and sincere promoter of my theoretical audacity. Danny Barreto has always been there for me when it counted. Bonnie Honig taught me more about mortalism than anyone, and so much of this book springs from lessons I had with her. I cannot write without hearing the voice of Katy Vernon, always a mentor and always a friend. Lisa Diedrich is both the real and imagined interlocutor for this book; your words open and end it, and I wrote this hoping it could live up to your brilliance.

The COVID-19 pandemic shut down too many things, but I was fortunate to find a brilliant group of friends in an online writing group: Mary Kate Donovan, Leslie Harkema, Catalina Iannone, Gabrielle Miller, Martin Repinecz, Anita Savo, Jon Snyder, Amaury Sosa Velasco, Wan Tang, Sarah Thomas, and Nicholas Wolters. You cheered when I did, sent many emojis and gifs, and consoled and advised me through every worry, fear, and triumph as I completed this book.

Thanks to Chloe Johnson at Liverpool University Press for enduring my silence with patience, and for working hard when things were slower or more complicated. The anonymous readers of the book were thoughtful, generative, and kind in their remarks. The editors of the series and the copy-editors moved this book forward into reality.

My family has been vital to the spirit of this book, and our circle has grown and shrunk in the years that I have been writing it. My aunts Jennie and Sandy showed me what love could look like, even when I couldn't yet imagine it. My brother Jeremy and sister Jennie have been excited for my professional accomplishments and have offered warmth, humor, and care even when our experiences and worldviews differed. May our group chat continue, but may we use our phones a little less. My beloved partner Josh has endured a decade of book talk with good grace and wise advice that I should heed more often. He is the first to pull me out of the minutiae of academia, and I can't thank him enough for being there. I look forward to our next pizza night. My mother Geri sat down and filled out my first college application for me. It is too small to say that I would be nothing without her: I will be eternally buoyed by her endurance, love, and spirit.

All of my work exists because of my grandmother, Julia Garrison née Alvira-Torres. She taught me my first words in Spanish, and with that, opened up new worlds to me. My father, who passed away while I was finishing this book, worked through chronic illness his entire life. I learned of the power of stillness and thoughtfulness from him. I miss them both dearly, and I wish they could have seen this work completed.

To everyone named here, and everyone I foolishly forgot: you are all in this book.

Introduction: Feeling Sick

Illness affects us all, inside and out. We are preoccupied with the movements of our bodies through our environments, we dither over the invasive elements that infect or interact with us, and we worry about our predisposition to faulty genes or the likelihood that our bodies harbor malignant viruses or germs. Even in its purported absence, as when we promote health and wellbeing, we do so as a way to avoid sickness or to ameliorate the maladies we are already coping with. As such, we all live with illness, erratically and unpredictably exposed by our vulnerability to forces both external and internal. We don't think of our lives this way, of course. When we are sick, health is always just over the horizon, a state we will return to without fault; when we are healthy, it is the natural way of things, our purest state of being. We want to think of illness as anomaly.

It is not. Throughout this book I underscore the centrality of illness to modern ways of being and, in doing so, explore how popular imaginaries of life have been animated by wellness and physical vulnerability. Reframing the vitality of illness in this way recodifies our relationships to it, potentially upending its wholly negative connotations in the emphasis of what can be born from illness, or what it can produce. In part, such a move strikes against the belief that illness is just the absence of health, a bad byproduct of poor lifestyle; it also stakes a claim for the vitality of illness as a means to think through what it can do for us, and what we can learn from dwelling with—as opposed to overlooking or overcoming—our often sour relationships to our sicknesses and debilities. None of this is easy, of course, particularly when illness is real, sorely visceral, unpleasant, and painful. Recentering illness in life may also seem callous, a product of a blithely naïve (or naively academic) line of thought, one which ignores the crushing realities of illness and debility. Perhaps we don't want to fixate on illness because it's all we can do to survive it.

It is a fallacy, though, to think that illness will relinquish its hold on us just because we wish it so. In reality, it isn't health that is always over the horizon, but its lack—and eventually, entropy-bound as we all are, illness and infirmity are all we've got. In her acclaimed *Illness as Metaphor*, Susan Sontag famously called illness 'the night-side of life, a more onerous citizenship' before going on to say that 'everyone who is born holds dual citizenship, in the kingdom of the well and in the kingdom of the sick' (1990, 2). Although her ultimate goal is to discredit the metaphors impressed upon illness, to flatten them and arrive at an untainted understanding of the term in its fullest sense, these opening lines suggest otherwise. The imagining of illness as geographical space, an emigration into a dark land, does something significant to the concept: it places boundaries around the category of illness, ordering it into an inhabitable and politicized space. Sontag speaks of illness as geography, which ultimately is a metaphor for identity and an understanding of the connections we as citizens have to our own undesirable and undesired countries, the interior and exterior spaces where we come into contact with other bodies, germs, and pathogens. What we say about illness, then, highlights what is already at work in culture and language, a conceptualization of what occurs within the self and the body when confronted with the specters of disease, sickness, or debility. These metaphors subsequently exert themselves upon representations of illness, particularly in the earliest reports on the HIV/AIDS epidemic. By understanding how representation and metaphor are at once colluding and colliding with illness, we are able to better critique the ways that they delineate and uphold the shape of the social body, or how they work to embed patterns of sexual normativity as well as sustain new categories of personhood.

Our routine representations of illness thus keep us bound to a specific imagining of the way sickness works. That is, once they have been established, our notions of illness in general—and of certain ills in particular—encourage us to collect a discrete set of rules regarding their social and cultural meaning, who they can and cannot affect, and the social price of infection. This has particularly been the case with the HIV/AIDS epidemic, which has perennially revived global concerns about modern interconnectivity, social disparities, and the virulence of social and sexual contact. Initially emerging as a 'niche' illness that was thought not to affect so-called normal, healthy citizens, HIV/AIDS has deepened awareness of our susceptibility to tricky viruses and undercover sleeper cells even while significantly changing our relationships to our bodies, our blood, and our national and international communities. In the sort of journalism that is often produced in mass media (that is, sensational), reporters named HIV/AIDS 'the plague of the twentieth century' in countless articles, bestowing upon it a title that at once seemed hyperbolic and woefully inadequate in capturing the havoc it wrought. That this moniker came about in spite of the fact that more people have succumbed to cancer, heart disease, and even tuberculosis than from complications related to HIV/AIDS[1] would be puzzling if it were not for the powerful (and often damning) interplay between this illness and the cultural meanings it has accumulated.

Even its naming has been crucial in calcifying the most common perceptions of the syndrome. What is now known as AIDS (Acquired Immunodeficiency Syndrome) was rather infamously first called 'GRID' (Gay Related Immunodeficiency) by physicians in 1982, as the majority of initial cases struck the homosexual communities of San Francisco, Los Angeles, and New York. GRID was attributed to everything from sadomasochistic sexual practices to the use of poppers (amyl nitrate) during sex. Some months later, at a summit in Washington, D.C., the illness was officially given the name 'AIDS' by political and health officials. The discovery of what would be called the Human Immunodeficiency Virus (HIV) did not come until 1983, and it was not named as such until 1986. HIV is the retrovirus that, when left untreated, weakens the immune system to the point where it is susceptible to opportunistic infections and illnesses that are thwarted by otherwise healthy systems. When one's CD4+ T cell count is low enough and AIDS-defining illnesses are detected, the person is considered to have developed AIDS. A person with HIV may never develop AIDS, though the two are often considered to be synonymous. These things were, of course, not known in the earliest years of the epidemic, a fact which colored perceptions of HIV and AIDS and which still contributes to the slippery signification that equates one with the other. Writing about these years, additionally, means sifting through references to 'AIDS' which are sometimes meant to be 'HIV', or interpreting terms that were commonly accepted science (i.e. 'AIDS antibodies') that now have other names or meanings. To preserve original meaning, this book sometimes uses 'AIDS' in deference to its usage in the archival materials studied here, while at other key moments I have chosen to designate these as 'HIV/AIDS' to avoid the casualization of HIV as AIDS

1 This information is taken from the World Health Organization's 'The Top 10 Causes of Death' fact sheet (World Health Organization 2017), which details the top global causes of death in 2000 and 2015, and from the Centers for Disease Control's 'Leading Causes of Death' reports, which extend from 1981 to 1998 (Centers for Disease Control and Prevention 2015). I have kept their discrete categorization, although—and to be clear—many of these illnesses are not exclusive to HIV and can, in fact, result from a compromised immune system. The parsing of these illnesses from HIV/AIDS may be an attempt by the aforementioned organizations to separate out more clearly differing illnesses, although it also serves to maintain a sort of AIDS exceptionalism that exoticizes and mystifies its symptoms and effects.

which a moniker like 'the plague of the 20th century' derives), Diedrich also argues that epidemics be thought of as long histories. Such a move would have us rethink epidemics as requiring and challenging endurance, repeating and mutating intermittently, and extending backwards and forwards in time, far beyond epidemic origins or eradications. This line of thinking would, it should be noted, also bring about a revalorization of our relationships to illness—seeing sickness not as a cleft in time but part of time itself, not pressing itself against but into the rhythms of life. In short, as I have sketched above, rethinking the event of illness offers a means of recuperating its importance to daily life.

While she does not ultimately make the same claim as I do here, Diedrich's challenge to the conjunction of illness, thought, and activism in time allows her to

> account for the often indirect and unstraightforward relationships between very big things (environments, economies, histories, structures, ideologies) and very small things (genes, cells, viruses, conversations, gestures, and feelings) and between very fast things (a flash, an instant, a glimpse, a glance) and very slow things (the interminable, the evolutionary, the gradual, the glacial). (Diedrich 2016, 3)

Working from a similar approach, albeit with a wholly different subject, Lauren Berlant's *Cruel Optimism* considers the historicity of the global economic crises that swept much of the world in the late 2000s, and the responses of those who bore the largest brunt of them. In their book, Berlant lays out a way of thinking about the emergence of the historical present through the sense of living through a 'situation':

> a state of things in which something that will perhaps matter is unfolding amid the usual activity of life. It is a state of animated and animating suspension that forces itself on consciousness, that produces a sense of the emergence of something in the present that may become an event. (2011, 5)

This interplay between the 'usual activity of life' and the unfolding, materializing thing that may develop into something more—an event that disrupts those movements of life as we know them—bears some semblance to Diedrich's search through the knotty relationships between the fast and slow times of the events of illness. Primarily, I see both scholars as identifying the fundamental intimacies between times of crisis and ordinary life. Crisis is not always a rupture, they show—there are those who live closely and daily with crisis in a broad sense, just as there are others whose ongoing sicknesses preclude any sense of healthy normalcy whatsoever. I take some of this even further in this book, arguing that the AIDS epidemic (globally, yes, and particularly in Spain) be understood as much more than an illness of highly specific risk groups, areas, or practices, and that instead we think of the deep connections—both painful and productive—that it brings about, connections that tie us to others in critical vulnerability and precarity. By tracking the long, enduring time of the epidemic alongside its turbulent emergence, we may be able to see ourselves as bound together in tight but delicate ties, raw and open in our vulnerabilities.

In differing ways, both Diedrich and Berlant turn to the AIDS crisis as means of reconsidering illness-as-vulnerability; Diedrich focuses on the connections between queerness, illness, and activism, while Berlant considers the epidemic's place in defining a sense of what they term 'crisis ordinariness', which is used to argue that 'crisis is not exceptional to history or consciousness but a process embedded in the ordinary that unfolds in stories about navigating what's overwhelming' (2011, 10). Both moves see vulnerability (or precarity, another term that Berlant is particularly drawn to when discussing the repercussions of the 2008 economic meltdown) as part and parcel of human experience, especially when such experiences become entangled with illness.[4] There is much to be gleaned from that entanglement and from dwelling with one's own vulnerability, to loosely borrow from Judith Butler's phrasing in *Undoing Gender.*

The structures of feeling sick

The negative affect of illness has a profound impact on the way we live, whether it emerges out of a sense of vulnerability at a critical juncture in time, in anger or sadness at a diagnosis, or in the abiding feeling of being slowly crushed by pressures both economic and sociocultural. In their emphasis on the enduring vulnerability that is extracted from us in times of crisis, both Berlant and Diedrich take cues from Raymond Williams's *Marxism and Literature*, which spends some time identifying the development of the present from the past. As part of an emerging present,

4 I see both of these arguments as connected to the theoretical turn to mortalist humanism that has characterized some philosophical and political discussions in recent years. Broadly speaking, this line of thought advocates on behalf of a productive type of social, cultural, and political vulnerability that comes out of sustained contact with mortality, loss, and grief. Just a small sample of these texts demonstrates their disciplinary richness: *Undoing Gender* (Butler 2004), *Antigone, Interrupted* (Honig 2013), *Ugly Feelings* (Ngai 2007), and *On the Postcolony* (Mbembe 2001).

Williams discerns something he terms a 'structure of feeling', arguably one of his most famous contributions to the field of cultural studies. A structure of feeling, Williams reasons, is comprised of a number of affective engagements with relationships and thought that reveal 'meanings and values as they are actively lived and felt' (2009, 132). He further specifies that these relationships form a set, 'defining a social experience still in process, often indeed not yet recognized as social but taken to be private, idiosyncratic, and even isolating, but which in analysis ... has its emergent, connecting, and dominant characteristics, indeed its specific hierarchies' (2009, 132). By framing structures of feeling from within the development of the present out of the past, Williams highlights the importance of affect to the formation of temporal events. The feeling of one's participation in history in the making—a common sensation during epidemics, as noted above—is thus borne alongside a shared kind of 'practical consciousness of a present kind, in a living and interrelating continuity' (Williams 2009, 132). The distinction between thought and feeling breaks down, and the emotions of living through (or surviving, as Berlant relates it) an emerging historical event bleed into the way it can be ordered or codified logistically. The structures of feeling that begin to coalesce around the dawning present localize a distinctive sense of living through a special moment in time and history, an idea that is only verifiable once it is already over.

So much of what becomes apparent in the alignment of Diedrich, Berlant, and Williams's work is just how the structures of feeling surrounding the onset of the AIDS epidemic define and delineate a particular moment in time. In the chapters that follow, and in the materials that come out of this period in Spain, I find common threads of resentment, anger, confusion, fear, pride, love, and more; I see groups form and dissolve under the crushing weight of enduring an epidemic; and I note just how often temporality is brought to bear as a means of understanding the fleeting nature of life and the long fight for civil rights and social justice. I view all of this as the snapshot of a moment, a looking back at the structures of feeling of AIDS that comprise these early years of the epidemic. I further see the event of AIDS as a project of looking backwards and forwards, naming moments that have already gone by, but which still blossom into the present and future.

In relation to the potential of understanding these early years of AIDS as a particular structure of feeling, Gregg Bordowitz has worked to develop Williams's ideas further by advocating for a 'queer structure of feeling' that is formed around the relation between 'how heterosexist oppression attempts to contain queer sexualities, and how queers fight oppression by forming communities. Thus, a queer structure of feeling can be described as an articulation of presence forged through resistance to heterosexist society' (2006, 49). Bordowitz's development of the queer structure of feeling seems designed to combat the isolating effects of AIDS within global LGBTQ communities, a method of linking together generations despite (and in some ways, through) their decimation from illnesses related to HIV. In that sense, Bordowitz claims that a queer structure of feeling is fundamentally 'a set of cultural strategies of survival for queers' that 'describe a continuity in the structure that traverses a number of generations' (2006, 49).[5]

It is, of course, impossible to maintain that AIDS is exclusively a gay or queer person's disease, and I make no such claim as this here, despite its repeated appearance in the cultural materials of the early 1980s; I am, however, attracted to the intergenerational time of Bordowitz's queer structure of feeling, which pushes back against the loss of friends, parental figures, icons and more by reconfiguring what count as connective ties. Most importantly, that reconfiguration is laden with the negative affects produced by resistance, struggle, pain, and illness as much as it is brought forth through good sex, joy, and the pleasures of friendship. Establishing a queer structure of feeling that blossoms out of negativity, illness, pain—a model of being that can live with, not against, the daily slog through a time of a crisis—opens up possibilities for connective ties with others in moments when we normally think of them as breaking down.

Bordowitz methodologically develops the concept of the queer structure of feeling through a collection of essays on the AIDS epidemic titled *The AIDS Crisis is Ridiculous*. In order to understand better just what this queer take on Williams's work might mean for Spain and in the case of visual cultures surrounding AIDS, I want to only briefly examine a couple of moments from two of these essays. In the titular essay, 'The AIDS Crisis is Ridiculous', Bordowitz writes of a sexual fantasy he has of one of his artistic idols. In this fantasy, the pair have sex without a condom. As Bordowitz explains:

> My fantasy reveals that, unconsciously, I think that AIDS is the legacy I have inherited from the previous generation of gay men. It is difficult not to blame past lovers for my HIV infection, regardless of the fact that

5 It should be noted that Bordowitz's elaboration of what might possibly count as a queer structure of feeling has a very deliberate recuperative stance within queer liberation politics, especially as he writes that 'cultural work can be considered within a queer structure of feeling if self-identified queers produce the work, if these producers identify the work as queer, if queers claim the work has significance to queers, if the work is censored or criticized for being queer. A particular work is queer if it is viewed as queer, either by queers or bigots' (2006, 49). As seen here, I honor Bordowitz's original outline of a queer structure of feeling even as I crack it open by incorporating the queerness of illness.

> I know that no one is to blame—my lovers or myself ... The hardest thing I have had to accept is that there is no reason that explains AIDS. There are historical, material conditions that create a situation of crisis, but there is no reason why some people die, why some get sick, why I am infected. There is no reason, but there is meaning. My experiences are filled with meaning. (2006, 49)

As he reasons, the 'meaning' of Bordowitz's experiences connects him directly to an older generation of gay men through illness. He struggles with this legacy, this connection to the queer past, even as he gives himself up to it in fantasy, losing the prophylactic that divides the flesh of one body from the other. He fights this connection, or wants to, but ultimately must recognize that it affords him a sense of belonging through infection.

In his essay 'Boat Trip', Bordowitz examines even more explicitly the queer ties that bind him to the members of his HIV support group. Told as a series of journal entries narrating a trip that the group takes together, Bordowitz tells of lazy days on the water, collective drug trips, casual flirtations and angry run-ins, and the tedium of spending a little too much time with a group of acquaintances. One of the underlying themes of this essay, in fact, is the group's somewhat tenuous connections outside of their shared serostatus. Bordowitz anxiously spends time wondering if he will be able to form a bond that 'will transcend this, if our union will be justified by something more than each individual's need for support. Our love for each other, perhaps' (2006, 100). Certain moments of euphoria bubble to the surface, bringing a familiar feeling 'as if I've been in the company of all of these men all my life', like they are 'older male relatives who remain at the table after the women have removed the dinner dishes' or a 'group of buddies passing joints in parked cars overlooking scenic points' (2006, 100). These sentiments are in turn broken by the fear that some of their interpersonal relationships 'focus on death in ways that interfere with our enjoyment of life', essentially preventing them 'from being present in the moment, enjoying experiences' (2006, 100–01). He eventually recognizes somewhat glumly that there may be no great take-away from this trip, no moment when the group becomes anything more than one that is organized to cope with each other's deaths (2006, 109).

Both of these narratives tell complex stories about the desire for belonging in the midst of a destructive, contentious pandemic. What Bordowitz seeks in both is a model for surviving and thriving in which relationships come about because of illness but are simultaneously able to transcend it—a productive framework for intergenerational relationships that allows for something more to come from illness than the sense of being crushed slowly underneath the weight of one's mortality. It is unclear if this ever happens for him, although I hold that the struggle in itself for these relationships reveals how nuanced they are, how inflected with profound meaning and affect; this in turn suggests that the queer structures of feeling formed in the midst of illness can stretch and bend, allowing for a range of connections within something that is almost only ever considered a cataclysmic destroyer of health, social connections, and meaningful ties to others.

In the chapters that follow, I turn to the elasticity of structures of feeling in the early years of the AIDS epidemic in Spain in order to open up questions surrounding origin stories, identification with and against illness, representations of blood and sexuality and their interactions, and much more. I see Bordowitz's stories as revelatory to understanding the long time of crisis and illness, tracing out strategies that in turn bring about new ways to live and endure the long time of chronic crises. It should be clear, as it was for Bordowitz, that some of the relationships produced out of such structures of feeling are just as laden with pain and failure as the common experience of living through illness itself. Still, I am pointing to the fact that something new emerges in these early years of AIDS in Spain; it is alternately a sense of living through history, a gesticulation away from sick groups, a banding together in illness, a reactionary abandonment of hope, and a revolutionary turn toward the future. It is through illness—through HIV/AIDS—that this potential is brought about.

The utility that I find in Bordowitz's work is not entirely shared by Diedrich, who writes that his queer structure of feeling attempts to turn 'a structure of feeling into a survival strategy' (2016, 50), that it 'overinstrumentalizes the term and the cultural work it does', and that it produces the fundamental error of reducing the social to fixed forms (2016, 48). For Diedrich, Raymond Williams's original concept describes 'how cultural productions ... capture forming and formative processes without making them into formed wholes' (2016, 48). Seeing Bordowitz's concept as fixed and wholly formed, Diedrich underscores the ongoing materialization of the present from the past as it was originally emphasized by Williams, stressing the innately 'private, idiosyncratic, and even isolating' natures of a structure of feeling, which ultimately wind up feeling a little queer themselves (2016, 49). Rather than offer up a way to fight the oppression of queerness and attempts to contain it, as he imagines his queer structure of feeling to do, Bordowitz's description of the boat trip is instead 'about embarrassment, sadness, and unease about relations in the present moment and yet also hopefulness for the future: a structure of feeling rather than a fully realized strategy for surviving AIDS' (Diedrich 2016, 50). The attempt to formulate a survival strategy through the queer structure of feeling, in Diedrich's account, displaces Williams's original concept by creating something fixed out of something fluid; the failure of Bordowitz's strategy, further, means that in lieu of supplanting a structure of feeling, Bordowitz recreates it in the expression of living through the momentous present as it is still in process.

Diedrich is quite right to point to the failures and halting successes of Bordowitz's examples, which never fully become the idealized versions of themselves, especially as the author himself imagines them. Yet is precisely this failure that opens up the queer structure of feeling into something more than what Williams envisions. Through Bordowitz's work, we can distinguish a potential for understanding the world on the basis of sometimes unsatisfying or painful attachments and interconnections, and as a series of intergenerational exchanges that malfunction and sputter out at odd intervals. Bordowitz searches for an explicitly queer articulation of Williams's concept (that is, one formed on the basis of a specific sexuality confronted with AIDS), and in doing so he attaches prescriptive ideals about what it can look like. The intermittent ability of his relationships and attachments to live up to his vision of the queer world is, I claim, precisely what brings it about. This queer structure of feeling is therefore intimately tethered to bad affects and good, to illness and AIDS; it ruptures relationships and forges new ones, making uneasy, joyous, and ambivalent alliances. Working within the queerness of AIDS (which is enacted both through and outside of queer sexualities) forces an unexpected shift in Williams's concept in ways that are not immediately present at the outset.

In many ways, what I am getting at tilts closer to a structure of feeling *sick*. That is, as I have elaborated here, sickness has the potential to (and often does) fulfill many of the things that Bordowitz imagined of queerness: it stretches our sense of time's duration, inflects our relationships both destructively and productively, and breaches the discrete sense of one's self. In this imagining, then, I see a slide between illness and queerness that AIDS in particular makes patently felt. Diedrich herself toys with the reciprocity between being sick and being queer, developing this interplay into a way of 'doing sickness' and 'doing queerness':

> Illness queers identity categories, and it queers relationships between individuals, communities, and even nations. If we consider queer not in terms of a particular identity—that is, not as a form of being but as a mode of doing—then we begin to expand the affective and effective possibilities of the concept... What might it mean to do queer rather than be queer, and how might this doing create new forms of not only queer sexuality but also queer love, in this case within the particular domain of the politics of health and illness? (Diedrich 2016, 22)

Queer love, as Diedrich suggests here, is but one possibility for making queerness do more. The purported failure of Bordowitz's strategies of survival (read here instead as intermittently successful) taps into another one of the possibilities of queerness, which is that it is often made to work through loss, grief, and negativity. What Bordowitz imagines within a queer structure of feeling is its explicit linkages to queers suffering with AIDS; in emphasizing the threads that already tie queerness to illness, however, I want to gesture toward something even greater than this, a means of understanding the early years of the epidemic that go beyond a zero-sum understanding of loss and life. In the way that things like time, pain, love, and sex are rewritten by illness, transmuted virally into something more than the sum of their original parts, I see this era of AIDS as vital to our understanding of the way we relate to ourselves and to each other.

S.I.D.A.

The structure of feeling, as Raymond Williams conceived it, is intimately connected to the practices of recognizing and adjusting to the emerging historical present. In Bordowitz's reformulation, the adjustments to the historical present (and presence) of HIV/AIDS can feel like failing, can fall apart, and can be ruinous to one's own body or health just as easily as they may bring about new relationships, sexual pleasure, or happiness. Bordowitz makes clear what has already been keenly felt by many: that living through a present that has been infected by illness can make us feel bad, like we are tethered to bad relationships, subject to bad days, and at the cruel whim of bad immune systems. As I will insist throughout this book, however, the sensations that come out of the failures of feeling sick are nonetheless also fettered to strategies of coping and survival. The potential of illness to slide queerly between failure and success—even intermittently, alternating painfully between one and the other—ties together history, illness, and sex in ways that are both discomforting and tender.

In this introduction, I have turned to Bordowitz's early writings as both theoretical framework and as an example of art that struggles to narrate meaning in an emergent crisis. In the following chapters, I examine a number of films, flyers, news reports, and cultural ephemera from Spain that similarly attempt to understand the history happening all around them. At times the messages in these objects are incoherent, and in other moments they talk across each other—discordant voices attempting to communicate something vital, a sort of understanding of the present that is only beginning to coalesce and become visible. Williams writes that there will inevitably be differences in the perception of the historical present since it is neither fixed nor formed but still in flux. The heterogeneous identity positions of those living through and/or surviving the event itself also create huge perceptive differences of the event.[6] These variances highlight the distinct formal irregularities of structures of feeling, which for Williams are only barely decipherable in their newness:

> It is primarily to emergent formations (though often in the form of modification or disturbance in older forms) that the structure of feeling, *as solution*, relates. Yet this specific solution is never mere flux. It is a structured formation which, because it is at the very edge of semantic availability, has many of the characteristics of a pre-formation, until specific articulations—new semantic figures—are discovered in material practice: often, as it happens, in relatively isolated ways, which are only later seen to compose a significant (often in fact minority) generation: this often, in turn, the generation that substantially connects to its successors. It is thus a specific structure of particular linkages, particular emphases and suppressions, and, in what are often its most recognizable forms, particular deep starting-points and conclusions. (2009, 134, emphasis original)

Williams's insistence that we see structures of feeling as balanced on the edge of understandable semantic meaning and incoherence is particularly insightful when considering the explosion of information emerging from the early years of the HIV/AIDS epidemic: news reports speculated wildly, rumors circulated on talk shows and debate programs, physicians published in journals of limited circulation, and governments tentatively (at best) pushed out safety guidelines. None of this is precisely what Williams means when he speaks of a structure of feeling, which is tied to cultural production and the narratives it can imagine; still, examples such as these set the conditions under which stories of living through and against AIDS are produced.

A structure of feeling sick, as I've outlined it above, queerly links illness and sex while claiming failure and loss as productive and even dynamic elements of change. The narratives that are generated in such upheavals capitalize on new metaphors, repurpose existing ones, and cauterize feeling

6 Given the theoretical framework of *Marxism and Literature*, Williams is clearly more attuned to the differences that social class enact upon the emergent narratives of the present (2009, 134). It bears noting that I see a host of other factors—race, gender, and sexuality, in particular—as similarly responsible for the bifurcating stories produced in narratives of feeling sick in and during the global HIV/AIDS outbreak of the 1980s.

and affect as powerful descriptors of historical events. In Bordowitz's work, feeling sick at once questions and allows an intergenerational struggle for understanding, which we will see echoed in some queer cultural objects of this period in Spain; in other narratives in Spain and beyond, feeling sick can actually look sicker, sadder, or less hopeful. The expression of what AIDS looks like in this period differs wildly, as we will see in the texts and objects examined throughout this book.

By way of example, in the 1985 song 'S.I.D.A.' by the Spanish punk band Peor Impossible, HIV/AIDS is explored as a socially and psychologically devastating event that nevertheless provides space for reevaluating one's identity formation. As one of the earliest artistic responses to AIDS in Spain, the song exists as a 'pre-formation', as Williams writes, of an articulation of the linkages between illness and the self, health and others, and the increasing paranoia and hysteria of AIDS. The song opens with a funky bass line and the quick, repeated percussive sounds of a shaker, which bear no small sonic resemblance to the chitter of a locust or grasshopper. The result is a sound that is both ominous and upbeat, a low throbbing bass wrapped around the punctuating noise of something like an insect, a bug in your ear. The lyrics—half sung, half spoken—tell the story from the perspective of an unnamed, ailing character: 'No me encuentro nada bien / Oigo voces en la sombra / Oigo el grito de la niebla / Ululando por ahí' [I don't feel at all well / I hear voices in the shadows / I hear the cry of the fog / Howling around out there].[7] First describing the sensation as that of feeling unwell, the narrator goes on to describe how he hears whispers and howls emitting from ominous shadows and fog. Being 'unwell', then, is more than a physical state of sickness but a complete immersion into illness, a sense of being uneasily surrounded by something sinister. A sudden perspectival shift, however, turns from inward preoccupation to outward defiance, addressing a presumptively non-sick listener: 'Yo no soy el asesino / de tus sueños escondidos / Tengo alergia de tu histeria / Yo vengo del más allá' [I am not the killer / of your hidden dreams / I'm allergic to your hysteria / I come from the great beyond]. The narrator's manic slide between illness, fear, and defiance suggests the experience of illness as dissociative, uncontrollable, and more than a little threatening; for that reason, and even as he is sickly fearful of the shadows, the narrator is accusatory, lashing out at the hysterical reactions of the people he encounters. Denouncing their fear of his ability to kill their 'hidden dreams', he tears into the hypocrisy of those who are afraid to live as freely as he has, refusing to accept any sense of blame or shame for his illness. His sense of complete otherness—privy to otherworldly whispers

7 Unless otherwise stated, all translations are mine.

and vulnerable to uncontrollable physical responses—leads to the ecstatic exclamation that he comes from the great beyond, no longer fully human but something more. The tangible and intangible feelings of being sick thus collapse into something greater than both, an uncontrollable body thrust outside of itself by illness.

The music of the chorus shifts from the steady percussion and bass to a punk frenzy of guitars and synthesizers as the members of Peor Impossible shout in unison: '¡¿Quién estoy?! ¡¿Dónde soy?! ¡Qué terrible sensación!' [Who am I? Where am I? What a terrible feeling!] The query is immediately followed by the repeated cry of '¡SIDA!' [AIDS!], a shouted response that serves as both answer and epithet. The linguistic reversal of the expected formulation of the verbs 'ser' and 'estar' here suggest confusion, impermanence, and the mutations of illness; that is, by using 'estar', a verb that is largely indicative of passing states and transient situations, '¿Quién estoy?' asks who I am now, who have I become, and intimates that I am under a constant state of flux. Likewise, '¿Dónde soy?' fixes the character in space, binding him to a permanently locked place; phrasing the question in this manner asks where 'I' am able to exist ('Where can I be who I am?') and what specific locations might allow for my being. The primal scream of 'AIDS!' in response to such existential queries is the answer to who and where the narrator is as much as it is a frustrated cry into the dark, another howling voice in the wind. This is to say that AIDS is at once the culprit behind these sensations and the very channel by which they are possible—a terrible sensation of ecstatic force, an untethering of the self that disassociates one's humanity in exchange for a connection to something outside of space and time.

At least, these are some of the interpretative possibilities offered in 'S.I.D.A.' The necessarily subjective experience of illness means that actual experiences differed wildly as people struggled to describe living with HIV/AIDS; what is more, the momentous sensation of living through an emerging event gave rise to narratives that teetered on the edge of semantic sense and even usefulness. 'S.I.D.A.' organizes itself around the feelings of having AIDS at a particular moment in time when there was so little sense to the epidemic, and its metaphorical flailing offers up impotent rage and a picture of shattered communities just as much as it reorganizes selfhood under illness and imagines a powerful, communal cry of togetherness. The message need not be repeated, rational, or even possible to serve as an affective snapshot of a specific moment in time and to offer up a structure of feeling sick in Spain in the early years of AIDS, a feeling in which connections break down as often as they endure.

Viral states

In the chapters that follow, I find similar narratives which furnish a micro-history of affect in the early years of the AIDS epidemic in Spain by attempting to narrativize what it means to feel sick. That these histories might differ or disagree only speaks to the mutability of illness and queerness, a powerful demonstration of how their elasticity affects someone living through the historical event of an epidemic. By considering the micro-histories of AIDS (the personal, individualized, and at times contradictory histories of the epidemic) alongside the larger macro-history of the illness in Spain, I hope to resist a pat narrative of the way HIV/AIDS played out in the country; instead, the varied accounts reflect what it is like to struggle, to lose, to celebrate, to grieve, and to live and die in an age of transition and upheaval. The stories, films, news programs, and ephemera found in the following chapters trace out a queer feeling of illness that neither embraces permanent loss or pain nor good health and happiness.

As I have noted, this argument—of a historical moment in which illness is bound to transition, and which stutters between good and bad so blindingly fast that the difference is nearly imperceptible—runs counter to the broadly accepted histories of this period in Spain. That is, the temporal proximity of the 1978 democratic constitution and the HIV/AIDS epidemic binds the two together, interlocked such that democracy energizes the global lines of commerce and transit that help transmit illness, and illness in turn gives voice to fears about the increased interconnection of people, goods, and cultures. Lina Meruane, writing on the explosive impact of the AIDS epidemic in Latin America, frames the epidemic in part as a problem of mobility: 'Unlike the epidemics of the past, this syndrome and the narratives around it have crossed the world, connecting organic, geographic, political, and cultural territories as well as a range of disciplines' (2014, 11). Although neither its communicability nor its mobility are as virulent as is made out here, Meruane is right to note just how capitalism has provided fruitful pathways for viruses. In particular, she writes that 'the decreasing cost of travel and the appearance of new communication technologies that had not been available to previous diseases were part of the long process of capitalism's structural and institutional transformation that began at the end of the nineteenth century' (2014, 11). The move toward democracy in Spain was intimately tied to its Europeanization and role in the European Union (then known as the European Economic Community), which in itself was a move toward a more globalized and interconnected Europe. In light of this, Spanish democracy was meant to exploit all of the things that globalization vis-à-vis full European integration could provide. Meruane rightly sees the promises of globalization at that time as almost wholly idealistic:

> There was a dream of a current of riches that would *flow* globally, in all directions (in the worst-case scenario, the excess of capital would trickle fluidly down—that is, toward the poor) and where wealth would cross borders that were more and more unnecessary, even irrelevant, and reach every corner of the planet... The fluidity of the new institutional structures and of capital would be joined by the fluidity of personal communications and of movement, eventually eliminating differences and their segregating effects. (2014, 14–15, emphasis original)

In a similar move, José Ángel García-Rodríguez, a professor of microbiology and parasitology at the University of Salamanca, opened the 1984 school year with a lecture that set apart the transmission cases of the European West from the Communist bloc on the basis of their economic systems. Describing the documented HIV/AIDS cases of (what was then) Czechoslovakia and Germany, he states that 'la actitud oficial del bloque comunista establece que el SIDA al igual que el herpes constituyen enfermedades propias del capitalismo' [the official attitude of the communist bloc is that AIDS, as well as herpes, are diseases of capitalism] (1984, 29). García-Rodríguez immediately counters this assertion by criticizing 'la falta de libertad en la que se desenvuelve la vida en estos países' [the lack of freedom with which life is carried out in these countries], which he sees as a challenge to health and the dissemination of knowledge (1984, 29). Invoking freedom as exclusively coupled to capitalism—and pointedly not found in communism—García-Rodríguez casts the global flows of resources and capital as good and beneficial, and in so doing he marks competing socio-economic systems as unknowable, sick, and oppressed. He is, of course, not alone in linking capitalism to integration and freedom, particularly in this time period in Spain. In fact, the portrayals of the Spanish transition to democracy that have solidified in popular imagery have, until recently, largely played into this romanticized vision of the possibilities of greater economic integration with global capital. Regardless of the nuanced discussions around democracy that took place at the time—from conservative backlash or progressive disappointment to, eventually, broad disillusionment—the 1978 constitution stood out as a hopeful transition to a better world.[8]

8 Though strong and forceful critiques of the Transition have been around for as long as the Transition itself (and even before it was even named as such), popular discourse has until recently been largely positive. This was in part due to the broad

Although the democracy is largely considered to have fully solidified after the failed coup by Antonio Tejero in 1981, the health scares and epidemics of the 1980s dramatically recalibrated public perceptions regarding cultural interconnections, national wellbeing, and the idealized hopes pinned onto increased social and economic globalization. Jesús de Miguel and David L. Kirp have noted this as a trend in Spain, in fact, writing that 'the system of public health in Spain is built on reforms brought about by wars and epidemics, from the 1855 cholera epidemic to the Spanish Toxic Syndrome' (1992, 171). The pathways to modernity proffered by globalization, then, can also be seen as transmission routes that allow for increased reliance on foreign blood reserves, queer tourism and exposure to new sexual identities, and a renovated drug trade allied with certain anarcho-punk sensibilities. These routes of transmission, expanded as Spain further opened its commerce and cultures to Europe and the West, would soon be tied to the marginalization of the so-called risk groups of HIV/AIDS: hemophiliacs, homosexuals, and intravenous drug users. As I discuss at length in Chapter 1, this is not to suggest that these groups should in fact be considered dangerous, inherently risky, or prone to bad practices, which is how they were almost uniformly represented in the early years of the AIDS crisis, nor that the increased flows and transmissions of globalization inevitably contributed to the epidemic. Instead, I am pointing to the ways in which certain institutional structures allowed for increased and easier transmission—and that blame, if any should be placed, belongs to those who allowed the disease to slip into the populace in favor of increased profit.

Regarding the AIDS epidemic as one of modernity in Spain highlights its local specificities and illustrates just how these differ from the global pandemic. The nature of epidemics is such that state borders and boundaries are at once reified and erased, a paradoxical way of seeing that lays bare the constructed nature of borders under neoliberalism while also affirming their innate importance. Noting how 'microbial indifference to boundaries is a refrain in both scientific and popular writing about emerging infections',

support for King Juan Carlos I during the Transition (from both sides of the political spectrum) as well as state control of the media, which restricted aspects of what could be publicly said through its platforms. More recently, with the increasing revelations of fiscal corruption within the Spanish monarchy, the rise of certain progressive social movements, and the proliferation of meaningful political parties beyond the Partido Popular (PP) and the Partido Social Obrero Español (PSOE), there has been a more critical and vocal re-evaluation of the 'regime of 1978'. To name only a selection of these: Acevedo (2012), Baby (2018), Kornetis (2014), and Whittaker (2020) all provide counterpoints to the more positive narratives of the transition to democracy in Spain.

Priscilla Wald goes on to quote Richard Krause, who writes that 'like science, emerging viruses know no country' (qtd in Wald 2008, 33–34). Wald also draws attention to the 1992 report of the Institute of Medicine's Committee on Emerging Microbial Threats to Health, which opens by noting that HIV/AIDS 'surely should have taught us, in the context of infectious diseases, there is nowhere in the world from which we are remote and no one from whom we are disconnected' (qtd in Wald 2008, 34). This is a faint echo of Susan Sontag's work, as seen earlier; in *Illness as Metaphor*, Sontag spoke of illness itself as its own country, one that could be stepped in and out of, and in *AIDS and its Metaphors*, she writes that 'the AIDS crisis is evidence of a world in which nothing important is regional, local, limited; in which everything that can circulate does, and every problem is, or is destined to become, worldwide' (1990, 180). Even in 'S.I.D.A.' by Peor Impossible, as we have seen, the person with HIV/AIDS (and by association, the disease itself) sees himself as coming from a great beyond—an unnamed, unbounded, and metaphysical 'somewhere else'.

The immateriality of national borders to viruses and bacteria creates a unique dilemma when studying localized reactions to epidemics and disease. That is, an epidemic like HIV/AIDS makes visible the global connectivity between a specific group, country, or region and the rest of the world, and the movements and flows of increasingly connected populations allow for strategies of resistance to be shared and information to be disseminated. Nevertheless, the array of differences (cultural, political, economic, and beyond) between individual actors means that no strategy or treatment can be applied equally, and that autonomous responses will inevitably occur. The HIV/AIDS epidemic is thus both global and extremely specific, ignoring national borders even as it prompts highly localized medical, political, and cultural responses.

This problem is akin to what Murray sees in the meanings given to blood and blood donation:

> Blood alone will not magically solve the problem modernity poses—how to keep the language and the practice of solidarity alive in an era when our mobility and communications blur the distinction between neighbor and stranger. We can witness the calamities befalling people half a planet away or listen to strangers reveal intimate secrets, perhaps while family members sit silently nearby. (1991, 237)

Unlike some of the more optimistic impressions of this modern era of mobility, Murray sees the global pandemic of HIV/AIDS as responsible for rupturing fragile local structures of community and endangering solidarity (1991, 233). The potential for intimate, local communities is thus traded for technologies of mobility and mediated social connections. In this formulation, the contradictory global and local characteristics of the HIV/AIDS epidemic poison local communities and further set forth the boundaries of the domestic and the foreign; for this reason, among others, we see a rush to police certain categories of citizens as members of so-called risk groups. The global transmission routes that allow for the viral spread of illnesses cast the infected person as external to the local community, tainted by a foreign agent.

Consequently, and even if some borders are often summarily dismissed in both popular and epidemiological accounts, some specific geographical types are reified. In the accounts of emerging infections, Wald writes that illness is often seen as both 'a product of global modernity and an indication of a return to a primitive past, a world not only without antibiotics ... but one in which medicines offer treatments that were often no more effective than prayer and witchcraft' (2008, 44). Ascribing the geographical origins of HIV/AIDS to Haiti and Africa led to an explosion of racist imagery that further catalogued an entire continent as dark, primitive, and deadly. This type of imagery—and the insistence on the temporal and geographical markers of the AIDS epidemic—is clearly corroborated in the earliest news reports on AIDS in Spain, which often cast HIV as a foreign and exotic illness, as detailed in Chapter 1. For Wald, such specific localization means that there is often a 'geography of disease' (2008, 44) that marks the types of narratives that coalesce around the origins of illnesses and epidemics.

These earliest years of the AIDS epidemic, then, show a pandemic that is represented as a global, borderless problem which is nevertheless tainted by its perceived and real origins and which produces localized reactions and repercussions. Examining the early years of AIDS in Spain is a way of acknowledging the specific shape its outbreak took and of understanding the particularities of local responses in an age of increased interconnectivity. Rethinking the portrayal of the Spanish transition as underwritten by illness, in turn, asks that we reflect on the governing assumptions and narratives about progress and productivity. If Spanish integration with Europe was brought about in tandem with illness, what else might be touched by the slow spread of being and feeling sick?

I began this project thinking that I might uncover some forgotten or waylaid truth about the HIV/AIDS epidemic in Spain, and as a result might better give a complete story of how things actually happened. Turning to wonderful but incomplete film and text archives in Barcelona and Madrid, visiting the non-digitized television archives of RTVE in Madrid's Prado del Rey suburb, and haphazardly finding items and documents on eBay and other auction sites has revealed what many already knew—that the HIV/AIDS epidemic upended lives so dramatically and thoroughly that many historical traces have been lost, blurred, and misplaced. I often went looking for archival materials in Spain only to find something entirely different—a flyer for a San Francisco bathhouse, a German condom kit distributed in bars, a pack of AIDS trading cards from California in the early 1990s. At times the archives just weren't there; that is, neither in the place I expected them to be, nor as plentiful as they might have been, or just missing. This noticeable absence—a suggestion of what could have been or what was but which can no longer be found—owes to lack of government funding, the stigma surrounding the epidemic and its risk groups, and the sudden loss of so many people. What has survived tells a partial story.

In a similar fashion, many of the texts produced in the earliest years of HIV/AIDS in Spain attempted to make sense of the spread of the virus in the United States or of AIDS as a global phenomenon, and thus missed some of the most crucial moments of its increasing virulence in Spain. These texts are nonetheless essential to this book and have been touchstones for understanding this chaotic and turbulent moment in history: the essays of Alberto Cardín, the work of Juan Vicente Aliaga on art and AIDS, and the writings of Ricardo Lorenzo and Hector Anibitarte, Paul Julian Smith, Alberto Mira, and more. As I write in Chapter 1, some of my initial surprise upon reading these authors is not the silence surrounding AIDS at the time, but how much was being said, and how hard certain groups and people were fighting to be heard.

Loss, silence, and pain are key elements of this book, as important as the texts that have survived and the celebrations of life they often contain. By framing Bordowitz with Peor Impossible earlier in this introduction, I have worked to piece together narratives that emerged in the historical event of illness and which describe what it can look like to live with and survive HIV/AIDS. These examples, as well as the archival fractures and gaps from the early years of AIDS in Spain, speak to a struggling narrative in pre-formation, a queer structure of feeling sick found across texts and objects and even in absentia. The historical situation that is HIV/AIDS, in turn, reiterates the impact of the epidemic in Spain as the country underwent its transition to democracy and deepened its connective ties to the world. The resulting smatterings of narratives and stories, discursive survivors of a devastating epidemic, describe the affective event of how illness makes history, and how it can become baked into the very sociopolitical life of a country like Spain.

These stories begin with the first reported cases of AIDS in Spain. In Chapter 1, I examine how medical literature and news reports worked to craft a national outbreak narrative of the illness. I draw from Priscilla Wald's

Contagious: Cultures, Carriers, and the Outbreak Narrative (2008), which describes the complicated process of ascribing meaning to origin stories of illnesses and the very real repercussions that these meanings create. She locates what she calls the 'outbreak narrative', which follows 'a formulaic plot that begins with the identification of an emerging infection, includes discussion of the global networks throughout which it travels, and chronicles the epidemiological work that ends with its containment' (2008, 2). In this way, even the index cases (those cases which are used to identify and mark an emerging outbreak) are folded into a narrative that is carefully shaped to fit governing ideals as well as orient popular opinion. Working with Wald's conceptualization of the outbreak narrative, I trace out a similar pattern in the initial reports on the index cases of Spain: a homosexual man who died in late 1981 and two hemophilic adolescents who died a little over a year afterwards, in the early months of 1983. Though their story came out after news of the first case, the media almost exclusively focused on the case of the brothers, amplifying it as the index case for Spain. Thus, and as suggested in this introduction, the outbreak narrative in Spain is laced through with prevailing ideals of healthy and sick bodies and communities, along with irregular archival practices that allow some documents to be buried and forgotten while others are sensationally made into headlining news reports.

Turning to Paul Julian Smith's *Vision Machines* (1996), de Miguel and Kirp's 'Spain: An Epidemic of Denial' (1992), and Patricia Keller and Jon Snyder's 'Encounters with the Unsightly' (2011), I negotiate previous accounts that seek out the origins of AIDS in Spain in order to draw attention to the tendency to fall in line with the desire for a unilateral, singularly true outbreak narrative. Working within the accounts that these texts offer for the outbreak narrative, I challenge existing ideas about how the crisis came about, how it spread, and what effect this flow of (mis)information had in the past and toward the present. I return to a structure of feeling sick to signal just how the conceptualization of an outbreak narrative seeks to organize the present from within, an impossible task when we consider how history is never known until it has already been concretized. That is, the outbreak narrative codifies events into discrete, compartmentalized stories that obey an existing national mood; a structure of feeling sick, the affective response to living with illness during an ongoing moment in time, is instead propelled by the paradoxical frustrations, hurts, joys, and victories of loss. By pointing to the inconsistencies of the outbreak narrative—which nonetheless has a very real effect on Spanish culture and Spanish lives—I signal the breaks in the unified, crafted story of the origins of AIDS in Spain. In the last half of the chapter, I analyze the first Televisión Española (TVE) special news reports on AIDS, 'Alarma: El virus que viene de California / Alarm: The Virus that Comes from California' (1983) and 'SIDA: La enfermedad de los 80 / AIDS: The Illness of the 80s' (1983). By way of a close reading of these two reports, I locate visual clues and images that signalled the Spanish outbreak narrative; by pushing back against this narrative and opening up its cracks further, this chapter rewrites what it means to think of the origins of the epidemic, which were at once deeply global and highly localized.

As part of the global origin story of AIDS, certain so-called 'risk groups' were denominated. These groups were thought to be made up of those who were, by virtue of their sexual or physical proclivities and needs, most particularly susceptible to HIV (or 'the AIDS antibody', as it was known at the time). Although it is no longer common practice in medicine to refer to risk groups (instead, the focus is on risky practices or behaviors), their establishment set aside communities of sick bodies from the public at large, falsely promoting a sense of safety among those who fell outside of risk. The remaining three chapters work from within the common structure of the risk group by analyzing representations of hemophiliacs, homosexuals, and intravenous drug users, respectively. This structure is also actively called into question, however, by the incorporation of objects and events that continuously underscore the interconnected nature of these groups. In short, I make use the framework of the risk group as a tactic that undermines the very utility of the construct as epidemiological practice.

Chapter 2 is focused on representations (and their lack) of hemophiliacs in the AIDS outbreak in Spain, who saw themselves as wholly apart from the cases of homosexuals and drug users with AIDS. Returning to two specific origin cases of AIDS in Spain, the pair of young hemophilic brothers who died in 1983, this chapter examines how the figure of the child becomes a plot point that is used to depict the hemophiliac with AIDS as more innocent and pure than others with the same illness. I turn to Kathryn Bond Stockton's *The Queer Child, or Growing Sideways in the Twentieth Century* (2009) and Sarah Wright's *The Child in Spanish Cinema* (2013) which, in varying ways, consider the place of the child in popular film and media coupled with the commonplace appeal to futurity and innocence that such representations bring. In thinking of the representation of the future, I also work with Lee Edelman's *No Future* (2004), which has polemic yet productive uses when considering how drastically AIDS affected the hemophiliac population of Spain. By way of case study, I examine a televised interview in the special news report 'SIDA: Crece la alarma / AIDS: The Growing Alarm' (1985) with the father of an adolescent who died of AIDS. I also return, briefly, to images of child hemophiliacs in the first televised report on AIDS in Spain, 'Alarma: el virus que viene de California / Alarm: The Virus that Comes from California' (1983). Addressing further representations of children in danger from sex, blood, or the otherwise aberrant monstrosity of adulthood, this chapter analyses two episodes of the much-loved television health program *Más vale prevenir* (1985 and 1987), the science program *Generación 800* (1985), and the variety show *El domingo es nuestro* (1987). Together, these programs and reports shape an image of AIDS in its earliest years as intimately tied to youth and childhood, the face of the future in Spain, even as they work to safeguard the normalcy and health of that figurative future. The end result is an attempt to rewrite the damage wrought by illness for a segment of the population, even as others were left behind in the past.

The final section of this chapter looks at the portrayal of blood as both life substance and disease carrier, or, as Dorothy Nelkin writes, as 'the apogee of purity and the nadir of filth; cited as both the basis for unity and justification for war' (1999, 2). By examining the representation of blood and blood products in medical literature on hemophiliacs with AIDS, the laws regulating blood donation and blood product purchase in Spain, and the imagistic representation of childhood in the magazines put out by the Spanish Hemophiliac Association, I contend that the belief in the purported virtues of national blood ties toxicity to foreignness and infects childhood with monstrosity. Calling forth innocence and futurity in this manner does something queer to childhood, forcing its reader to imagine death, mortality, and blood alongside conceptualizations of health and nationhood. I return to the structure of feeling sick here, proposing that such a move allows us to re-center difference into the national promise of a normative future for all.

Chapter 3 begins by deconstructing the common representational practices that pair homosexuality with AIDS. As in previous chapters and in the introduction, I trouble many of the practices from these early years that utilize easy notions of what the LGBTQ community is and was, and to whom it belongs; in contrast, and as Lisa Diedrich writes in *Indirect Action* (2016), I turn instead to the ways in which 'illness queers identity categories, and it queers relationships between individuals, communities, and even nations' (2016, 22). As such, this chapter begins with a brief consideration of the place of homosexuality in the years after the dictatorship, particularly the ways in which institutional control over the LGBTQ community was still administered and maintained, despite the presumptive legal freedom provided to queer people. This is to say that the long-held blending of illness and queerness together meant that both categories and subjects had become normalized, infected by each other and unable to be easily divided. I thus track how certain sexualities became re-criminalized through linguistic, metaphorical, and medical practices, even after their post-dictatorial legal decriminalization.

Turning to a range of cultural products and ephemera, this chapter sees a recuperative queer movement toward overt sexuality at a time when it was stigmatized and seen as a threat to the Spanish state and its people. I turn to the ephemera produced by gay collectives like FELGT (Federación Española de Lesbianas, Gais, y Transexuales / Spanish Federation of Lesbians, Gays, and Transsexuals) and by a number of anti-AIDS committees across autonomous communities, which emphasize issues such as community engagement, education, safe sex, and resistance to governmental stigma and community pressure. I also study the performance piece 'SIDA da' (1984) by Las Pekinesas, who use humor and deconstructive wordplay to defuse the queer panic behind the epidemic and to infuse it with playfulness, sexuality, and a little bit of chaos. Lastly, this chapter examines two educational pamphlets made by famed *Movida*-era artist Nazario which toy with raunchy and explicit sexuality in order to promote safe sex among men who have sex with men. Examining the LGBTQ community's responses to the pandemic alongside the constant fears of queerness-as-illness sees an explosive cocktail of queer humor, sexuality, and anger blasting open the silence of the early years of AIDS.

In Chapter 4, I turn to one of the most maligned risk groups of AIDS, that of intravenous drug users. A disparate group made up of women, men, members of the LGBTQ community, and children born to drug users, this chapter examines the stigma attached to intravenous drug users in the media of the time and the isolating and crumbling spaces they were forced into. In considering how these groups are made to flow together—not existing as a coherent group but forced into one by a blend of governmental, medical, and legal practices of the time—I analyze the cultural portrayals of drug users with AIDS as integral voices in the production of a structure of feeling sick in Spain.

This chapter examines the convergence of drug use, the prison system, drug dens, and drug users in order to think through the links between crime, AIDS, and drugs. As in Chapters 2 and 3, I see illegality, law breaking, sexuality, and monstrosity as key components to the representation of AIDS in the early years of the epidemic. In this case, however, these components form a unique blend with powerful repercussions for the treatment and response to AIDS in Spain. That is to say that in Spain, unlike other countries, AIDS infection rates and new cases were frequently tied to drug use. For example, by September 30, 1985, drug users 'represented 8% of all European cases and were reported by nine countries ... Italy and Spain together accounted for 63% of the IV drug abusers with AIDS in Europe. Forty-five (49%) of the 92 Italian patients and 23 (37%) of the 63 Spanish patients were members of this risk group' (Centers for Disease Control and

Prevention 1986). In contrast, male homosexuals accounted for less than half of all known cases in Spain (hemophiliacs and drug users made up the larger percentage). In other words, despite the public perception of AIDS as a 'gay disease', AIDS and drug use were tightly linked in Spain.

The narrative that dominated, however, never underscored drug use as a key component in combating misunderstandings and misinformation about AIDS. Just as importantly, the outbreak narrative that developed around the illness never saw drug users as anything but deadbeats who refused treatment or help and were essentially lost causes. Documenting this narrative, I analyze news reports on drug users and prisoners, noting how the portrayal of different risk groups holds to a well-established dichotomy between those who deserved illness (homosexuals and IV drug users) and those who didn't (hemophiliacs, children, the public at large). In addition to primary source materials, I incorporate a range of cultural studies on drug use in contemporary Spain, including texts by Francisco Fernández de Alba, Juan Gamella, Juan Carlos Usó, and Tom Whittaker.

In this chapter I frame the problem as one of ruins; that is, the drug dens that were often made in the actual ruins of abandoned buildings, occupied and hollowed-out spaces of crumbling edifices, and in the ruinous lives that drug users were and so often are portrayed as living. I follow Tim Edensor's work on memories and ruins, which analyzes 'how the effects of the disordered spaces of industrial ruins can interrogate and contest the normative ways in which memory is spatialised in the city' (2005, 829). I take two particular sites of memory as culturally significant markers of HIV/AIDS, drug use, and incarceration: the Escuelas Pías ruins in La Latina and Carabanchel Prison. Both of these become exemplary ruins of HIV/AIDS, meaning that the ruins created alongside and by the illness are seen at once to be eyesores but erasable, objects to be bulldozed out of the narrative or physically razed. This is, of course, another way of saying the same for people with AIDS. Whether through the deliberate selection of a 'perfect victim' by the media, the solidification of communities as sexual predators, or the incarceration of the hapless reprobate, people with AIDS were codified and made to fit a crafted narrative of who falls outside the borders of the community and state.

In the conclusion, I turn to an unfinished film by one of Spain's most prolific and mythologized B-movie directors, Jesús 'Jess' Franco, who wrote and directed the first 'AIDS film' to be made in Spain in 1986: *SIDA: La peste del siglo XX* [*AIDS: The Plague of the Twentieth Century*]. The film captures the mystery and terror surrounding AIDS in 1986 in sensational ways, particularly in its portrayal of the virus as a malevolent, androgynous alien force bent on sexually conquering the world. Franco's fantastic vision of the illness wrapped up fatal sexuality, mysterious transmission methods, and fears of queerness in a frenetic package, serving as a compact example of the polyvalent voices vying to be heard at this time.

This book focuses on the earliest years of AIDS in Spain (1981–1987) precisely because the sense of history-in-formation is so profound during this period. By 1987, there was both a test for HIV antibodies and early therapeutic approval for the drug azidothymidine, or AZT, both of which would change the narratives and the possibilities of living with HIV/AIDS drastically. The pre-treatment era, characterized as it was by uncertainty, was thus markedly distinct from an encroaching era in which substantive medical intervention was finally possible. By way of conclusion, I offer some thoughts on the developing sense of what HIV/AIDS was beginning to mean in Spain—the range of reactive feelings to the threat of HIV/AIDS that gave way to any number of attempts to mitigate anxiety, cope with loss, laugh away the threat, or ignore its potential. Of course, some of these attempts ran counterproductive to progressive activism and the effort to curb the increasingly desperate fear toward the perceived risk groups of AIDS. As I note in the conclusion, a structure of feeling sick isn't always productive, nor does it always get things right—it is an expression of one's relationship to the present, an attempt to feel one's way forward in time. The richness of such expressions has its own importance, though, and understanding how we felt around so blindly in the past can offer a way forward through the present.

CHAPTER ONE

Origins

To solve a mystery or a crime, you need to locate your villain. In cinema, the culprit is sometimes earmarked early on, distinguished from a few other potential rogues carefully, while at other times he or she is left on the sidelines as a few red herrings momentarily draw away the viewer's attention. The end result is ultimately the same, and the villain is revealed in all of his or her dastardly glory, reveling in the slaughter and harm of innocents and heroes. Ultimately, most audiences hope, good somehow triumphs. In the types of viral illnesses that can affix themselves to large populations, there is often a similar need to locate the bad guy, the one who brought whatever scourge we're facing to our shores and to our lives. Most particularly, as in the moralizing discourses that have surrounded AIDS and HIV since its early years, locating the illness's epicenter has taken on the frenzy and fervor long reserved for outsmarting Moriarty, staking Dracula, or tossing water on the witch.

If the pairing of classic cinematic villains with the initial patients of epidemics seems a little disingenuous or, worse, bogus, it should. In *Illness as Metaphor*, Susan Sontag points out how the mediation and metaphorization of illness have warped not only common perceptions of sickness but specific ills themselves, weaponizing metaphors and investing natural processes with meanings that extend far beyond their physical effects. As illnesses are increasingly mediated, reported on and made known, their images revert to distorted perceptions of diseases which further warp the realities of illness. Consequently, illnesses like typhus, Ebola, or AIDS have been thoroughly mediated, made into metaphors for social ills and cultural malaise and shot through with Manichean narratives. The representations of Mary Mallon, Mabalo Lokela, and Gaetan Dugas (three of the most recognized index cases of the epidemics above, respectively) have likewise been invested with a range of cartoonishly evil attributes. Thus Mary Mallon becomes the filthy and careless Typhoid Mary; Mabalo Lokelo becomes the guileless and backwardly barbaric stand-in for Africa as cradle-of-diseased-life; and

Gaetan Dugas becomes the promiscuous and willfully dangerous Patient Zero. Such transformations scrub the humanity from the people infected with these illnesses, reducing them to little more than ego-driven desires. This action of stripping away the thin skin of morals, in turn, reveals the filthy, villainous germs that are believed to lurk within us all.

As recounted in popular media, illness origin stories often take the event of sickness and transform it into a story of good and bad events, heroic doctors and villainous germs, and martyred innocence and murderous passions. Underneath these stories often lurks a dense sort of morality that emphasizes loaded concepts like cleanliness, goodness, and safety. Being physically clean or using safe sex practices may actually prevent the spread of illness, but overloading the significance of cleanliness and safety with moral undertones has damning effects for the way we imagine health and wellbeing. This is perhaps seen most evidently in the occasional use of the word 'clean' to informally denote someone who is HIV-negative. This usage implies interior cleanliness, which in turn becomes akin to a moral purity and is often connected to one's goodness. What is unspoken, yet acutely understood, is that being seropositive is 'unclean' or 'dirty', and thus both HIV/AIDS and the person living with it are cast in exclusively negative terms.

As is true in many societies, the rich histories of illnesses in Spain—and their ways of dealing with concepts like contagion, exclusion, and expulsion—meant that the initial treatment of AIDS would likewise be heavily metaphorized.[1] These metaphors, in turn, ascribed specific (and often negative) meanings to certain people, events, and groups over others. The origin story crafted by Spanish media culture around HIV/AIDS, then, put forth a specific way of understanding the illness that was seeded in social mores. As the illness spread, this metaphorized origin story took root in fears of contagion, isolating specific people, groups, and practices as dangerous, unsafe, and unclean, and organized a linear narrative out of the chaos of sickness. It has subsequently informed all responses to the HIV/AIDS epidemic in Spain. By examining the construction of that narrative,

1 A range of academic texts have studied the history of metaphors of contagion in connection with minority communities in Spain, the exile of these, and/or the confluence of health and national identity in Spain from the early modern period onward. To name just a small selection: *Communities of Violence: Persecution of Minorities in the Middle Ages* (Nirenberg 2015), *Medicos escritores en España, 1885–1955: Santiago Ramón y Cajal, Pío Baroja, Gregorio Marañón y Antonio Vallejo Nágera* (Sosa-Velasco 2010), 'El movimiento higienista español ante el 98' (Campos-Marin 1999), *Visions of Filth: Deviancy and Social Control in the Novels of Galdós* (Fuentes-Peris 2003), and *The Return of the Moor: Spanish Responses to Contemporary Moroccan Immigration* (Flesler 2008).

this chapter looks to understand the 'beginnings' of AIDS in Spain, the news reports that sought to create a specific national meaning for the illness, and the formation of 'risk groups' out of everyday citizens.

Uncovering the index case

Initial news reports in Spain were quick to underscore the foreign nature of AIDS, pointing first to the Californian coast's hedonism and ultimately to Africa, purported hotbed of disease, as worlds away from the newly minted Spanish democracy. In 1983, when AIDS was first widely reported as having arrived in Spain, it was almost immediately dismissed as a disease that only someone else could catch—hemophiliacs, homosexuals, or heroin users.[2] The very first cases of AIDS were identified in 1983 as two young hemophiliacs, brothers who died in Andalucía after receiving transfusions of infected blood coagulant from the United States; later, the medical report of a patient from late 1981 would resurface, a gay man who had traveled to the United States and Turkey and who had become infected after several sexual affairs that deviated from his purportedly 'stable' single-partner relationship (as the medical report of the time was quick to note). As the numbers of people with HIV/AIDS in Spain grew and patterns of infection began to emerge, the media fell into the near universal practice of denominating so-called risk groups that isolated them from the public at large; as a result, AIDS was passed off as a niche illness, one that could only strike a certain subset of the non-normal, deviant, or hedonistic.

This brief summary is clearly only part of the beginnings of HIV/AIDS in Spain, as this book seeks to make evident. The search for the index case of AIDS in Spain was an attempt to 'get at' the illness, to understand its emergence and foresee its effects. As time passed and as global patterns of illness emerged, this search gave way to calls for better treatment and care for Spanish people living with AIDS alongside the pursuit of a clear national response to the epidemic. But the belief in an identifiable origin story for AIDS, one that could organize panic into hope and provide a sense of futurity

2 This would become a fairly formulaic process for early news reports on AIDS across the globe. The identification of what came to be known as 'the Four Hs' of AIDS—heroin users, homosexuals, hemophiliacs, and Haitians—incorrectly isolated these groups as those who would solely be affected by HIV/AIDS. Not all of these 'Hs' were universally applied, however: the initial outbreak of AIDS among a small group of Haitians in New York City led some United States physicians to speculate that the illness's most likely route of infection was from Africa; Spain's geographical proximity to Africa but relative racial homogeneity in the early 1980s, on the other hand, precluded Haiti as a potential transmission route.

within morbidity, remained embedded in the treatment and mediation of both HIV and AIDS for years to follow. Attempts to organize these first years of AIDS in Spain into an understandable narrative, consequently, are often invested in origin stories, in pinpointing a cause, and in locating the index case.

The establishment of the index case—a person who is identified as the originating case of an illness or epidemic—is one of the first actions made to determine the severity of an epidemic, and it has taken on deep symbolic weight in the way an illness is represented within a culture. Much of its loaded meaning is due to the fact that this epidemiological act transforms a person into a case, covering up the individual and reducing them to a string of recognizable symptoms that coalesce into illness. This is clearly not to say that establishing the index case is a purely damning process to the public or to isolated individuals; on the contrary, it is vital to public health authorities and can help quell diseases by determining biochemical origin, potential rate of infection, and likely contact routes. The steps to establishing what is called a 'case definition' of an illness is related mainly to these initial cases: upon receiving news of the first reported case through public reports or medical personnel, public health officials seek clinical information from lab work, negotiate a timeline and geography for the case, and trace potential contacts of the outbreak.[3] These findings establish the seriousness of the illness and the protocol for its treatment. As such, the medical importance of the index case is undeniable.

The organization of the findings from index cases into a linear narrative, however, frequently filters an ostensibly neutral medical case through personal beliefs and prejudices. In *Contagious*, Priscilla Wald refers to this process as the construction of an 'outbreak narrative'. For Wald, the standard outbreak narrative follows 'a formulaic plot that begins with the identification of an emerging infection, includes discussion of the global networks throughout which it travels, and chronicles the epidemiological work that ends with its containment' (2008, 2). Such a narrative may be scientific, journalistic, or fictional (2008, 2), or even a combination of

3 This is a simple sketch of the general protocols that have been set forth by the Centers for Disease Control and Prevention (CDC), which are similar to those of the World Health Organization (WHO). In Spain, the Ministerio de Sanidad, Servicios Sociales e Igualdad [Ministry of Health, Social Services and Equality] oversees the national coordination of programs and regulations as well as the investigation of transmittable illnesses such as HIV/AIDS. For further information on the history and current status of Spain's 'Plan Nacional sobre el SIDA' [National Plan for AIDS], see the Ministry's dedicated webpage at https://www.mscbs.gob.es/ciudadanos/enfLesiones/enfTransmisibles/sida/home.htm.

all three; that is, to put it clearly, the description of an index case may have a medical origin even while promoting an outside agenda. In their investigations, Wald goes on to say, epidemiologists decide what constitutes a specific group or population, define wellbeing for the general populace, and create connections between the disease and the purported lifestyles and habits of different groups (2008, 19). Such criteria form the basis for epidemiological outbreak narratives, ultimately, and 'import cultural assumptions that are substantiated by the authority of medical science and the urgency of a public health threat' (2008, 19). In this manner, the work of the public health official and epidemiologist is hardly immune to the dangers of narrativizing or making metaphor of illness.

The meaning ascribed to the index case often mutates even further in public discourse. Reporting an index case isolates an illness, but it may also socially ostracize a person, implicitly designate a racial or ethnic group as 'tainted', and encourage a problematic dirty/clean designation for certain individuals or communities. When Wald writes that the outbreak narrative formed from the index case 'fuses the transformative force of myth with the authority of science' (2008, 33), she is indicating just how specious its potential may be in public discourse. Outside of its medical significance, the search for the index case transforms into another process altogether—it is a deliberate act, one that betrays a need to fashion a clear, linear narrative out of what is often thought of as the chaos of illness. It also establishes an origin point, creates a timeline, and begins the act of assigning blame for the incursion through the borders of immunity.

In this manner, the index case is at once medically useful and culturally hazardous: it singles out an origin point but almost immediately corroborates prevailing associations with an illness, deploying an outbreak narrative that continually mutates within a culture. This is most vividly seen in the creation of the term 'Patient Zero', which first appeared in journalist Randy Shilts's influential book on the origins of AIDS, *And the Band Played On* (1987). Condemning the disorganization and lack of governmental support for HIV/AIDS sufferers in its early years, Shilts turned up a single individual who would be made wholly responsible for the global pandemic: a French-Canadian flight attendant named Gaetan Dugas. Shilts extrapolated his evidence from a 1984 *American Journal of Medicine* article, which provided a contact trace of gay males with the cluster of opportunistic infections which had come to signal AIDS. In the *AMJ* piece, 'Patient O' represented the initial contact and transmissibility was noted between other patients in Los Angeles and New York (these patients would go on to become 'Patient 1', 'Patient 2', and so on) (Auerbach et al. 1984). These findings were based on an even earlier report in the June 18,

1982 issue of the *Morbidity and Mortality Weekly Report*, which highlighted a 'non-Californian' and his role in the emerging illness; amid the swirling numbers of patients and their illnesses in the *MMWR*, the non-Californian reappears several times in the contact wheel as having had sexual contact with several patients from across the country (Centers for Disease Control and Prevention 1982a). The non-Californian was referred to as Patient O, which was used to denote his origin as being 'Out[side]-of-California' (McKay 2014, 171). The misreading of the letter O as a zero led Shilts to mistakenly perceive a clear originating figure, the root of AIDS in the United States, and thus Gaetan Dugas would eventually be adopted by Shilts in a move that collapsed several narratives into one.

Shilts utilized this information to develop the nightmare image of Gaetan Dugas/Patient Zero as willfully deviant and obstinate in his refusal to limit sexual contact, a move that only serves to underscore a problem that emerges in many index cases of contagious epidemics—their villainous portrayal in popular media. This is not to say that the reports in the *Morbidity and Mortality Weekly Report* and the *American Journal of Medicine* did not contain their own extrapolations or inherent biases; in fact, Wald deftly shows just how these reports made logical leaps in the discovery of Patient O, notably in the fact that 'the numerous sexual partners reported by many people with AIDS ... combined with the lengthy latency period that the evidence increasingly demonstrated, would make it impossible to pinpoint an exact source even for most of the cases recorded on the chart' (2008, 229).

Journalistic, fictional, and even medical accounts of index cases tend to follow a familiar pattern in which the originating case is marked as a hybrid of the local and the foreign. This configuration of the index case is likely a result of the way that we view illness as a foreign attack on the sovereign soil of our autonomous individuality. Specifically, as Sontag has noted, the incursion of illness into one's physical body is often positioned as an attack from the outside, a non-native element that attempts to take down one's local, interior self. Wald writes that 'the inextricability of disease and national belonging shapes the experiences of both; disease assumes a political significance, while national belonging becomes nothing less than a matter of health' (2008, 67). Following Wald, this book operates from the position that illness is always politicized, just as national belonging is always already related to health and wellbeing. The figure behind the index case, as living representation of an illness or disease, is configured in precisely the same fashion. Consequently, someone like Gaetan Dugas was made representative of gay populations around the world even as he was continually presented as foreign and, worse, a domestic terrorist threat. Like the reports in the United States, the initial accounts on index cases in

Spain attempted to mark the disease as unique to particular risk groups and wholly foreign, as an outsider illness that attacked a select few domestically. The constructed representation of AIDS in Spanish culture of the 1980s, then, was a complex amalgamation of the foreign and the domestic; the result was a cocktail of stories that emphasized the strangeness, mystery, and exoticism of the illness over the actual facts and figures of an epidemic spilling over its borders.

Medical reports are not immune to the lure of the outbreak narrative either. As noted earlier, the first recorded medical case of AIDS in Spain originated in Barcelona's Vall d'Hebron hospital, and the physicians' report of the case was published in the March 6, 1982, issue of the medical journal *The Lancet*. Titled 'Kaposi's Sarcoma and Taxoplasma Gondii Brain Abscess in a Spanish Homosexual', the report notes the similarities in opportunistic infections between the anonymous Spanish patient and those in the United States. It goes on to describe the state of the patient: 'In October, 1981, a 35-year-old male homosexual was admitted with a 2 week history of fever, headache, and purple skin lesions on his trunk. Anorexia and weight loss had started 6 months earlier, and 2 months before admission the first purple skin lesion had appeared' (Vilaseca et al. 1982, 572). The account of the purple skin lesions paired with the reductive designation of 'homosexual' is more than merely descriptive—it is a deliberate move to link this patient to a global epidemic by means of coupling his sexuality to the now classic signs of Kaposi's sarcoma. In so doing, the *Lancet* report does far more than simply describe facts or symptoms—it interprets them, flagging a specific set of signifiers that conform to a rapidly emerging outbreak narrative of AIDS.

This outbreak narrative is further cemented as the report continues: 'Although he had a stable, one-partner relationship, during visits to New York in 1974 and Turkey in 1980 he had had sexual contacts with different partners. Over the 2 years before admission he had had repeated episodes of gonorrhea. He denied habitual drug use' (Vilaseca et al. 1982, 572). While the figure of the willful, deadly, and promiscuous Patient Zero would not be firmly established for a year or two more, its prototype is fully evident here. That is, in underscoring not only promiscuity but adultery, the patient is shown to abide by the sexualized stereotype of the gay man; the 'stability' of a one-partner relationship is thus traded for adulterous sexual pleasure, a sinful activity that is further underscored by the patient's 'repeated episodes of gonorrhea'. Yet how are we to define a relationship's stability: as monogamy, as the uninterrupted duration of a relationship, as emotional or physical commitment? How can a physician presume to measure this stability, except as a betrayal of her/his own moral partiality? The use of 'although', moreover, implies a logical contradiction that exposes the report's unquestionable belief in the wholesome nature of monogamy and the 'stable', faithful partner: 'although' he had a partner, the report says, he had sex with other people. In this manner, and while careful not to make a full pronouncement on the sinfulness of the patient's actions, the report makes its moral leanings clear.

The *Lancet* report does not suggest that the patient deserved these terrible illnesses or his subsequent death from brain abscess, but it does see danger represented in the homosexual community. This danger exists in the form of an encroaching physical epidemic—the purple lesions, the cancers, the strange influenza attacks—but also as an endemic sickness of careless moral permissiveness found in bathhouses, cheating partners, and rampant (homo)sexuality. In its final lines, *The Lancet* notes that 'reports of other European cases of opportunist infections in male homosexuals with or without Kaposi's sarcoma suggest that the international homosexual community as a whole is at risk' (Vilaseca et al. 1982, 572).[4] The international homosexual community was (and still is) at risk, yes, but so were (and still are) many other communities. Bracketing the disease to a minority group isolates the danger based on its initial index cases while also implying blame in some way, suggesting that there is something that this person or group is doing to bring about its own demise.

While the case of the gay man is a precautionary moral tale, a finger-wagging parable of rampant sexuality, the case of the hemophiliac brothers strains against this damning narrative. The recipients of infected blood coagulant, Juan Antonio and Diego de los Reyes Mesa contracted HIV/AIDS in Seville some time in 1982. Diego passed away in January 1983, while Juan Antonio died in April of that same year. The brothers were not officially confirmed as having had AIDS until May 1983, months after the onset of their symptoms. Yet as will be seen in the earliest special reports

4 Interestingly, the article that immediately follows this one in *The Lancet* also displays many of the same characteristics of the Spanish case. Ostensibly detailing the first AIDS case in France that bore similar symptoms to the global epidemic, 'Multiple Opportunistic Infection in a Male Homosexual in France' writes: 'The patient is a male homosexual, aged 38. His last visit to New York was in February, 1980, when, for the first and only time, he took "poppers" several times. He has never taken other drugs before or since' (Rozenbaum et al. 1982, 572). The moral framing of the report shows how invested physicians had become in correlating theoretically deviant sexual practices with the origins of AIDS; the association of the patient's trip to the United States with the contraction of his illness, as in the case of the Spanish man, likewise recurs to displaying AIDS as a disease both foreign and hedonistic.

on AIDS, the treatment of their story in the Spanish press was remarkably different from the description of cases among gay men at the time. As two of the first hemophiliac cases of the epidemic in Spain, Juan Antonio and Diego were seen as innocent victims of a terrible disease, two children who had died in the crossfire of bad medical practices and the spreading taint of a homosexual epidemic.

This does not mean that the brothers were wholly immune to the moralizing discourse that so often accompanied reports of index cases. In a May 5, 1983 article in *El País*, journalist Alfredo Relaño provides the curious note that the brothers were 'pertenecientes a una familia modesta que habita en una barriada periférica de Sevilla, el barrio de la Oliva, con altos índices de delincuencia y consumo de droga' [belonging to a modest family living in an outer suburb of Seville, the neighborhood of Oliva, with high rates of crime and drug use] (Relaño 1983). The inclusion of this information in an article that details their illness and contraction of AIDS would be curious if it did not yet again uphold the damning nature of what it means to be an index case. The explicit incorporation of drug use and crime into their story, particularly when neither boy was ostensibly involved in either, seems motivated to inspire either suspicion or pity over their background. The further description of the family seems designed to confirm their sad existence: 'El padre es un empleado de una central lechera y la familia se componía hasta esta tragedia del matrimonio y cinco hijos y pasaba estrecheces económicas. El mayor de los dos fallecidos, Diego, era sordomudo y tardó mucho en ser escolarizado' [The father is a dairy worker and, until this tragedy, the family consisted of two parents and five children and was facing economic hardship. The older of the two deceased boys, Diego, was deaf-mute and was slow to be schooled] (Relaño 1983). Despite its pitying tone and fundamental differences from the medical report on the anonymous gay Spaniard, Relaño's article begins to craft an outbreak narrative for Diego and Juan Antonio that moralizes and editorializes the story of those who contract HIV/AIDS. The focus on loose morals and risky practices in the medical report of the gay man is replaced with this article's correlation of poverty and sickness, and Diego and Juan Antonio are seen to be victims of a social sickness, rather than a moral or sexual one.

As will be seen in the contemporary televised news reports from Radio-televisión Española (RTVE), Relaño's focus on poverty mirrors the global phenomenon of 'Africanizing' the HIV/AIDS epidemic. Underneath Relaño's description of the brothers' origins lurks the threat of Third World poverty in Spain, a blight on a country which had only recently recovered its European, First World status. Pointing to a mythic, primordial origin for AIDS that stretches back to Africa is a way of displacing the domestic cases of an illness, signaling the exoticism of AIDS, and blaming an always removed other. This followed a larger pattern of representing the risk groups of gay men, drug users, and hemophiliacs as faulty, and their bodies as host to '"Third World" immune systems' (Wald 2008, 241), as Wald describes the popular view of the time. The boys' impoverished origins and their propensity for illness are consequently set side by side, and Diego's disabilities are read as a product of the family's poverty; the end result of this article and the *Lancet* report is the fabrication of two narratives which begin to sound eerily similar, and which propose that belonging to any of these marginalized groups (gay, poor, or sick) is a fundamental risk to one's health.

These stories of the anonymous gay man and the hemophiliac brothers serve as clear examples of the power of the outbreak narrative in popular culture. As index cases of AIDS, they defined the illness for a whole country, and intimated the risk believed to be inherent to certain groups and practices. Yet, and despite its appeal to journalistic, medical, and social communities, the index case is hardly an infallible structure to an epidemic's outbreak. As the near contemporaneity of these cases shows, HIV/AIDS was clearly not limited to one entry point in Spain, and its simultaneous documented appearance through sexual contact and blood transfusions suggests an unknown number of further avenues of transmission, potentially undocumented lives and deaths that passed without leaving institutional records (a point that is further explored in Chapter 4). Following the index case of an illness, then, may contribute to understanding one of the multiple paths an outbreak takes within a given populace, but it is scarcely the whole picture. As Wald writes of HIV's introduction into the United States: 'It is, in fact, unimaginable that if HIV entered the United States from without, it did not arrive in multiple hosts. Lack of documentation of the earliest cases and an unpredictable incubation period would make it impossible to pinpoint a single index case' (2008, 234). The same must be considered as we approach the myth of the AIDS origin story in Spain and the vilifying outbreak narrative that has shaped institutional and societal reactions to the illness.

Signs of the times

Despite the fallacious narratives they construct, and even after these index cases have been buried under years of further facts and figures, they still haunt the story. Such haunting has much to do with the political climate of Spain at the time. In *Vision Machines* (1996), Paul Julian Smith correlates public reaction to HIV/AIDS with the political atmosphere after Spain's transition to democracy. During the *Movida*, the artistic anti-movement of Madrid and Barcelona that gave rise to popular figures such as Pedro Almodóvar, Costus, and Alaska,[5] Smith notes that the political and cultural climate of the time seemed apt for a public discourse surrounding AIDS; indeed, he writes, 'the endemic weakness of the Spanish Right ... and the relative absence of populist, tabloid journalism suggested a certain consensus around public health policy and inhibited the grossest homophobic outbursts experienced in other countries' (1996, 102). Elsewhere, Jesús de Miguel and David Kirp find it 'surprising that AIDS should be so significant an epidemic in Spain' (1992, 169). Citing the association that AIDS in its first decade held with either 'prosperity and liberation (as in the United States) or with poverty and traditional sexual practices (as in Africa)' (1992, 169), they go on to list a range of features that would seemingly have hindered the spread of the illness within Spain: 'a low rate of homosexual contacts, a weak and divided gay community, strong social control over sexual mores, and a public health system ... that offers free medical care to almost everyone' (1992, 169). The dark years of the dictatorship behind it (in principle, if not truly in practice), Spain seemed ready to implement real change in the social and political policies that had held it back for so long. The first years of the AIDS epidemic in Spain, then, represented a moment for the country to assert its independence from the vestiges of the dictatorship and the cultural mores to which it had been bound.

Yet despite the theoretically welcoming climate in Spain in the early 1980s, the public discourse surrounding AIDS was often weak, misinformed, and—at worst—nonexistent. Smith claims that this silence stemmed from the transition to democracy and the shifting rules of representational politics: 'The representative democracy enjoyed by Spain, and the long, clandestine opposition which preceded it, have tended inadvertently but definitely to distance citizens from the public sphere and to delay the representation of new issues or communities in that sphere' (1996, 123). Citing studies by Juan Vicente Aliaga and Miguel G. Cortés, Smith describes just how the

5 As discussed in the Introduction, the definition of what the *Movida* was—including its ideals, its influences, and its legacies—remains contested in Spanish cultural studies, as evidenced in *Toward a Cultural Archive of La Movida: Back to the Future* (Nichols and Song 2014) and *Queer Transitions in Contemporary Spanish Culture: From Franco to la Movida* (Pérez-Sánchez 2007). Still, it is undeniable that the *Movida* helped shaped youth culture in Spain by promoting artistic production, providing an outlet for political dissatisfaction, and stimulating a burgeoning culture of liberated sex and drug usage. The relaxation of social mores regarding drugs and sex, in particular, would become particularly significant after the emergence of AIDS in Spain.

tactics that worked favorably during the decades of the Spanish dictatorship hampered public action in the new democracy:

> During the dictatorship, dissent could not be individual, but was rather highly organized... And since revolutionary struggle was channeled through a 'monolithic' Left political structure, then problems would inevitably be delegated to the appropriate representatives. While PWAs in the US felt obliged in the absence of social welfare structures to assume individual responsibilities, in a Spain which now enjoyed free and universal health care, there was no tradition of forming self-protection groups, pragmatically centered on single issues. (1996, 123)

De Miguel and Kirp have only a slightly different perspective on the effects of the transition from dictatorship to democracy, claiming that the 'four decades of Franco's repressive rule have left a legacy of popular distrust in Spain, not only toward the national government but toward officialdom generally' (1992, 173). In blaming an 'us versus them' mentality wherein the general public is at once suspicious of its government and has little power to influence policy, the authors also fault the lack of political representation afforded to society at large. The particular minority groups believed to be the primary index cases and carriers of HIV/AIDS, meanwhile, held even less political authority than the already disenfranchised Spanish public.

For the authors above, the resulting problem is one of visibility. AIDS cannot initially be seen, only then to make itself dramatically evident in the form of sarcoma, lesions, and physical deterioration. Likewise, the political transference of individual or minority dissent to organizations that represented the broad concerns of their constituents encouraged invisibility and isolated outliers (the emerging 'risk groups') in favor of a public that was theoretically safe from the AIDS outbreak. Thus, in place of a politically liberated society that was actively promoting the safety and health of its populace, AIDS revealed a profound systemic oppression amid the ruins of an old regime that haunted Spanish democracy.

Smith is right to point out the lingering political effects of the dictatorship's absence and the paradoxical silence of the liberated democracy as threats to Spanish public health in AIDS, just as de Miguel and Kirp do for the lingering distrust of government left behind in post-dictatorial Spain. Yet framing the outbreak in the familiar terms of invisibility fails to see the very deliberate, visible examples made of the Spanish index cases and their 'risk groups'. This is to say that AIDS wasn't exactly invisible; as early as 1983, as we have seen, the general public knew precisely where it was, who had it, and, according to the logic of the time, who would suffer from it. Although these groups would fluctuate as the decade progressed, the initial risk groups of heroin users, homosexuals, and hemophiliacs were constantly made visible in Spanish newspapers, medical reports, novels, films, and televised programs and debates throughout the 1980s. The threat to Spanish health was not one of invisibility, therefore, but of selective visibility.

This difference is more than mere semantics. Unlike the United States, where gay groups vocally and violently clashed with government representatives in order to receive recognition of the tremendous death toll of AIDS, the Spanish media seemed overly aware of its risk groups. The organization ACT UP (AIDS Coalition to Unleash Power) held protests on Wall Street and in Washington, D.C. in 1987 in response to the government's glacial response to AIDS;[6] yet as early as 1984, small groups of gay organizations in Spain were already being interviewed in news reports for RTVE, and the co-founders of the Comité AntiSIDA [Anti-AIDS Committee] in Madrid were routinely included in television debates and dialogues. This is not to imply that AIDS was a non-issue in Spain, to conflate visibility with acceptance, or to suggest that members of these risk groups weren't singled out in harmful and problematic ways—in fact, the visibility afforded to intravenous drug users and homosexuals in Spanish media was hardly benevolent, as we will see repeatedly throughout this book.[7] Despite the fact that homosexuals and drug users had been afforded certain freedoms by Spain's democratic government, which was 'committed, in principle, to progressive politics in the varied fields of sexual object choice and feminism, drug use and racism' (Smith 1996, 101), there still remained strong prejudices toward these groups in public sentiment. Indeed, as de Miguel and Kirp write, and in

6 As one of the first countries to mediate the HIV/AIDS outbreak, the initial (lack of) response to the AIDS crisis from the United States government is well documented. For further reading on this specific history, see *And the Band Played On* (Shilts 1987) and *How to Have Theory in an Epidemic* (Treichler 1999). For more information on the history and actions of ACT UP, see *Moving Politics: Emotion and ACT UP's Fight Against AIDS* (Gould 2009); *Melancholia and Moralism: Essays on AIDS and Queer Politics* (Crimp 2002); the online ACT UP Oral History Project (actuporalhistory.org); and ACT UP New York's archival website (actupny.com).

7 The omission of hemophiliacs here is intentional. As is explored in Chapter 2, the response to hemophiliacs who contracted HIV/AIDS was markedly different from the treatment accorded to homosexuals and drug users. This was primarily due to the method of transmission—hemophiliacs were portrayed as victims of AIDS, contracting the illness through tainted blood and not through a deliberate practice. The hemophiliac was therefore often portrayed as innocent victim, unlike the willful transmissions to which homosexuals and drug users fell prey.

spite of the 1978 decriminalization of homosexuality and the government-sponsored needle-exchange program a decade later, 'social attitudes have changed more slowly than the law. Even in post liberation Spain, opinion polls report, homosexuality and drug use are still condemned as sinful (though by lesser majorities than a decade earlier)' (1992, 174). Patricia Keller and Jonathan Snyder critique these new democratic policies even more sharply, finding that they 'fit neatly into troubling narratives that recast the disease as a collective sacrifice for new democratic freedoms of identity expression in post-Franco Spain' (2011, 93). In other words, one could now choose to do anything, but had to be prepared to suffer the consequences for those practices.

It is clear that the politics that guided national and regional Spanish health policies in these years were fueled by a dictatorial hangover that limited the democracy's potential. The treatment of AIDS was, for many, a problem of life and death—but it was also an issue that had deep political and social ramifications and pitfalls for the left-wing government in Spain. Mining the representational power of an index case, for that reason, could help shift policy in one direction or another as well as color public perceptions and media treatment of the illness. Unfortunately, however, the inaction and ignorance of the Spanish government and its health authorities led to their joint failure to take early advantage of the low case numbers in Spain; instead, the government remained content to pass AIDS off as a foreign disease that affected a select few, to organize it into camps of the marginalized, and to publicly boast of being safe from the disease's reach.[8]

Needless to say, such inaction had very real effects for the growing group of people with AIDS in Spain. In a timeline graphed by the HIV/AIDS organization SIDA STUDI, the slow response of Spanish officials to the initial outbreak in Spain—the lack of any response at all, really—is made painfully evident. Separated into three columns marked 'MUNDO', 'ESPAÑA', and 'CATALUÑA' ['World', 'Spain', 'Catalonia'] with a corresponding list of dates running their length, the timeline organizes the principal events of the global AIDS outbreak by year. For instance, in the 'World' column, alongside '1981', is an entry with the logo of the *MMWR* (*Morbidity and Mortality Weekly Report*) and a brief description of the report that is considered to contain the first mention of AIDS-related symptoms, '*Pneumocystis pneumonia* – Los Angeles' (Centers for Disease Control and Prevention 1981). There are similar

8 It bears noting that the decades since the onset of the HIV/AIDS epidemic have hardly taught us any lessons, it would seem, as many of these same mistakes would be repeated globally in the early months of the COVID-19 outbreak in 2020 and, at the time of writing, the nascent monkeypox outbreak of 2022.

entries for the first mention of AIDS in *The New York Times*, the date when AIDS was given its official nomenclature, and for the first cases of HIV/AIDS by way of blood transfusion. The 'World' column is filled with dates and brief factoids like these, marking the spread of the disease through populations and countries but with such an emphasis on the United States that considering it representative of 'the World' seems a little imprecise. The Spanish and Catalan columns for 1981 through 1983, in contrast, show a single, shared entry (SIDA STUDI 2011, 1).

The stark visual contrast between the three columns suggests the hybridized narrative belonging to epidemics such as AIDS. That is to say that the near emptiness of the 'Spain' and 'Catalonia' columns underscores the lack of national response to AIDS, yes, but it also links them to a unified, global origin story. The first few 'World' entries detailing the origins of AIDS, then, provide a context for the arrival of the illness in Spain while also displacing its origins outside of Spanish territory. The ultimate effect keeps the disease foreign—an already ever-present problem inherent to perceptions of illness—and occludes the necessary incorporation of AIDS as a threat requiring a unique, national response. The SIDA STUDI graph also evokes an origin story for a global epidemic that stretches back decades before its first official case, to 'el primer caso de una persona muerta a causa del virus en el Congo en 1959' [the first case of a person dead from the virus in the Congo in 1959] (SIDA STUDI 2011, 1). This proto-index case, 'primitively' located in time and geography, serves as a distant forefather to the cases of the 1980s; it remits the story of AIDS further back into the shadows, displacing the blame for the spread of AIDS to a source that is barely detectable.

The lone entry in 1981 for 'Spain' and 'Catalonia', meanwhile, is spread across the two columns and boldly highlighted in bright red, a sharp contrast to the light pink backgrounds of the columns. The visual effect draws the eye, underscoring its importance to the story of AIDS in Spain. The text itself presents a summarized version of the story of the gay man who contracted AIDS abroad:

> Octubre. Se diagnostica el primer caso en el Estado español en el Hospital del Vall d'Hebron de Barcelona. En aquel momento todavía no se hablaba de sida, sino que el equipo médico lo relaciona con un brote extraño de sarcoma de Kaposi y otras infecciones oportunistas que habían aparecido recientemente entre la población homosexual de Estados Unidos. (SIDA STUDI 2011, 1)[9]

9 'October. The first case is diagnosed in the Spanish state in the Vall d'Hebron Hospital in Barcelona. At that time AIDS is not yet talked about, but the medical team

As has been noted, the simultaneity of this report with the hemophiliac brothers calls into question the entire conceptual reliance on index cases in the first place. Further, SIDA STUDI's deployment of this story as Spain's index case requires a bit of narrative (if not chronological) sleight-of-hand, as the medical report was published in early 1982 but summarily lost or ignored for a little over a year; the national press, in the meantime, had devoted itself to the story of the hemophiliac brothers. The brothers, however, do not match up to the global reports of gay men dying in their thousands from the disease, nor do they represent the groups that were most affected by the illness (or who were continually referenced as being so in the form of 'risk groups'). Highlighting this particular index case, therefore, links Spain to the construction of a global origin story and contextualizes a timeline for AIDS within national and regional specificities. This final result is a constructed history of AIDS that displaces its origins so far back that we can never truly know them—even while it firmly maintains belief in an originating index case, the story of the people who brought the disease to Spain's doorstep.

Digital outbreaks

The very first special television report in Spain that focused exclusively on AIDS aired on RTVE on May 14, 1983, and was titled 'Alarma: El virus que viene de California' [Alarm: The Virus that Comes from California]. This report was shortly followed by 'SIDA: La enfermedad de los 80' [AIDS: The Illness of the 80s] in August of that same year. These reports were the first of their kind in Spain, and as such they dealt primarily with the theoretical and tangible origins of the disease, describing its at-risk populations and its methods of transmission in Spain and abroad. The titles of these reports are both evocative and meaningfully pointed: the 'alarm' of the first underscores the global tension (if not panic) that had begun to coalesce around AIDS while pointing a blaming finger at its perceived American origins; the second echoes scores of reports and headlines across the globe in defining AIDS as the illness of the decade.

Both reports aired in 1983, which points to the Spanish media's crucial dismissal of AIDS in its early years and its hurried attempt to catch up with the epidemic. As a reminder, the first cases of AIDS among gay men in the United States occurred in late 1980, and the report that linked the illness to

relates the illness to a strange outbreak of Kaposi's sarcoma and other opportunistic infections that had recently appeared in the homosexual population of the United States.'

(homo)sexual contact was published in June 1981. The medical report that connected the symptoms of the Spanish man to the rising phenomenon of AIDS, in turn, was published in early 1982, after his death in December 1981. So, from 1980 to the first report's airing, Spanish television was virtually silent on the topic, which contributed to the growing confusion and fear that surrounded the illness. Even as the first televised reports aired amid growing concerns that the illness had not only made its way to Spain but had begun to infect increasing numbers of the populace, they attempted to downplay the disease's contagiousness. AIDS had already firmly established itself as a prominent and deadly disease that affected thousands around the globe; what had changed, for Spain, was its national emergence in the form of reportable index cases. More so than the newspaper articles in *El País*, *ABC*, or *El Mundo*, these special reports gave a visual face to the epidemic in a powerfully visceral way. In this way, 'Alarma: El virus que viene de California' and 'La enfermedad de los 80' would cement an outbreak narrative for AIDS in Spain that would endure for well over a decade.

As the first report to deal specifically with AIDS as a global and national phenomenon, 'Alarma: El virus que viene de California' reifies popular beliefs in the disease's foreign origins while aiming for a working definition of what the disease means for Spain. This 'meaning' emphasizes the rise of AIDS cases among hemophiliacs in Spain, devoting particular care to the hemophiliac brothers. Lending special significance to these cases in particular forces the report to articulate a more-or-less clear distinction between the immune (or those who should be immune, by virtue of not belonging to a risk group) and the afflicted, dismissing the threat of AIDS for the majority of its televised audience.

The report opens with a brief introduction to AIDS: 'Esta enfermedad se denomina por el momento "Síndrome de Deficiencia Inmunológica Adquirida", o más brevemente dicho, "AIDS"' [This illness is currently called 'Acquired Immunodeficiency Syndrome', or its abbreviation, 'AIDS'] ('Alarma: El virus que viene de California' 1983). The host continues by carefully spelling the acronym out for the audience: 'A, I, D, S'. The recurrence to the illness's English etymology is altogether unsurprising. Despite the fact that AIDS had already received a more or less official Spanish translation in the form of SIDA (Síndrome de Deficiencia Inmunológica Adquirida), which is even used in the report, the failure to recognize the disease as anything other than a foreign illness speaks volumes about its perception as an outsider occurrence. AIDS, the report casually suggests, is a foreign disease that has begun to encroach upon Spanish territory; the as-yet unrecognized SIDA would be something else, a Spanish illness with a specific history and relevance to the Spanish public.

The report continues with a summary of the illness's history for the general public:

> Parece ser causada esta enfermedad por un virus ... no identificado pero que se manifestó de una manera activa en la costa oeste de EEUU en el año 1980, que se extendió ... lentamente por todo el país y que terminó alcanzando al continente europeo en el año también 1980, a finales de este año.[10]

Similar to the SIDA STUDI report, 'Alarma' highlights the mystery of AIDS's as yet unidentified virus, which also draws attention to its unexplained origins. The 'alarm' of the title, then, makes its first appearance in the threat of an unidentified, mysterious virus. References to the 'active' outbreak of AIDS versus its 'slow' transmission throughout the United States and Europe, in turn, both minimize the alarm and keep it ever-present.

The report cuts to a reporter who describes AIDS as a 'plaga gai' [gay plague], 'pneumonia gai' [gay pneumonia], and 'el síndrome de los homosexuales' [the homosexuals' syndrome]. Terrible as the nomenclature is, the organizational logic was similar to what was mapped out in the United States just a couple of years before, which marked AIDS as a uniquely gay disease. Even though the delay in its reporting meant that the global narratives surrounding AIDS had eliminated homosexuality as the sole spreader of the illness, the rising epidemic remained strongly marked as a 'gay illness'. Thus the early remarks in 'Alarma: El virus que viene de California' followed the unified, moralizing narrative already set up for the beginnings of AIDS: 'Nos encontramos ante una nueva enfermedad, ante un nuevo sindrome de oscura afiliación: El extraño sarcoma de Kaposi, de resonancias amenazadoras y bíblicas, se ha hecho dolorosamente popular como la plaga gai' [We have before us a new illness, a new syndrome with dark affiliations: the strange Kaposi's sarcoma, with its threatening and biblical undertones, has become painfully known as the gay plague.] The initial reference to the 'dark affiliation' of the disease is informed by its unexplained origins, but also by its suspected ones: both the unfathomable sexual acts that gay men commit among themselves and the dark continent of Africa, the primordial culprit for so many diseases. The purported 'strangeness' of the Kaposi's sarcoma lesions, meanwhile, recalls biblical plagues and in so doing correlates AIDS to sinful actions, hedonistic behaviors, and non-Christian communities.

10 'This disease seems to be caused by an unidentified virus ... that actively appeared on the west coast of the U.S. in 1980, which spread ... slowly throughout the country and ended up reaching the European continent also in 1980, later that year.'

The strangeness and mysteriousness of AIDS is delineated for a general viewing audience that, as the report implies, would never experience it. In other words, it promises a glimpse into a foreign world, one that is only faintly understood but heavily coded by moralizing narratives, while its audience remains untouched by its 'biblical undertones'. It works to establish an outbreak narrative, one that 'articulates community on a national scale, as it depicts the health and well-being of those legally within the borders of the state as a mark of their belonging' (Wald 2008, 33). Collapsing medical index cases with a narrative steeped in luminous Catholic virtues, this report defines who truly belongs to the healthy national community.

After this introduction, 'Alarma' jumps to images of people donating blood, which are quickly followed by a shot of the Hospital Virgen del Rocío, in Sevilla. The reporter somberly notes: 'En España, el primer brote conocido tuvo un trágico final con dos víctimas mortales: dos hermanos de 9 y 14 años, hemofílicos que fallecieron en Sevilla. El primero, el 11 de enero de este año, el segundo, el 14 de abril' [In Spain, the first known outbreak came to a tragic end with two fatalities. Two brothers, aged 9 and 14, hemophiliacs who died in Seville; the first, on January 11 of this year, the second, on April 14.] The tone of these opening remarks indicates the seriousness of the illness and, in decentering its perceived homosexual origins in the United States, the report attempts to create a case for understanding AIDS in Spain. That is (and despite the fact that there had already been at least one reported AIDS-related death within Spain's gay community), focusing on the threat to hemophiliacs offered a 'safe' outbreak narrative for Spain, one that dealt with media-friendly victims rather than with a group perceived as willfully hedonistic. The blithe references to AIDS as a 'gay disease' or as 'gay pneumonia', in turn, clearly differentiate the AIDS narrative in Spain from the illness's spread in the United States. As will be seen in Chapter 2, this was not a tactic that would hold in the long term, and the threat of illness to hemophiliacs diminished greatly as measures for blood testing became more and more stringent; still, 'Alarma' clearly works to provide a context for the illness, in some way, for the Spanish public.

The report continues by moving from its description of the first AIDS cases in Spain to aerial shots of New York. There are some shots of African Americans dancing, and light jazz music plays in the background. The visual move from the somber tones of the hospital in Sevilla to the bustling nightlife of New York draws a distinct line between the emergence of AIDS in Spain and the United States. The voiceover continues: 'El procedente del síndrome: de apariencia lejana. Se situaba hasta ahora en la costa oeste de los EEUU, con la sospecha de su existencia en algunas comunidades subdesarrolladas. Algo muy lejano, hasta ahora. Hasta hace poco, a fueron apareciendo casos en Bélgica, Inglaterra, Suiza' [The provenance of the syndrome, seemingly far away. Until now it was located on the west coast of the United States, with the suspicion of its existence in some underdeveloped communities. Something far off, until now. Until recently, when cases began appearing in Belgium, England, Switzerland.] The pairing of dancing African Americans in New York City with a voiceover that references the West Coast origins of AIDS seems a strange mismatch, and one that is easy to dismiss as a simple editing error or ignorance; closer inspection, however, reveals a complex overlay of presuppositions and beliefs ascribed to AIDS in the United States. References to the 'faraway' roots of the disease allude to the physical and cultural distances from California to Spain, while the shots of Black people dancing serve as visual shorthand for the even further away Africa. Citing the 'underdeveloped communities' suspected to host AIDS further suggests its presumed origins and contributes to the 'africanization' of the illness, even if the report itself denies such knowledge. The result is a highly charged pairing that—yet again—places an idea of Third World poverty alongside homosexual hedonism, providing an unspoken but powerful message that the blame for the epidemic belongs solely to these groups.

Establishing 'africanized' homosexuals as the primary culprits for the disease's spread throughout the globe and the impact of AIDS in Spain on the hemophiliac community, 'Alarma' looks to the origins of the disease. Referencing 'los orígenes nada claros del "síndrome de los homosexuales", otro de los apelativos asignados a la enfermedad' [the unclear origins of the 'syndrome of the homosexuals', another one of the names assigned to the illness], 'Alarma' utilizes a combination of skewed facts and moralizing discourse to confirm popular fears and beliefs regarding AIDS. In doing so, it reifies loosely grounded information into a clear outbreak narrative that damns the homosexual community of the United States: 'Parece ser que, al menos estadísticamente, ha partido de cierta promiscuidad homosexual. Siete de cada 10 casos de los originados en los EE. UU. correspondían a la comunidad gay masculina de aquel país. Era—es—un dato' [It seems that, at least statistically, it has stemmed from homosexual promiscuity. Seven of each 10 originating cases in the United States corresponded to the gay male community of that country. It was—it is—a fact.] The imploring call to the 'facts' of AIDS is meant to allay doubts as to the real culprits for the disease's global influence, but it barely masks its contempt for gay sexuality (promiscuous or otherwise). This is to say that this 'fact' is but one of the many facts about AIDS; highlighting its spread among gay men as a problem of promiscuity ignores the spread of HIV/AIDS among women, intravenous drug users, sex workers, Haitians, hemophiliacs, primarily monogamous homosexuals, and many others. The clarificatory slip from 'was' to 'is' a fact, meanwhile, insists on the continual threat that gay male sexuality allegedly has on an imagined—and otherwise healthy—public.

Ultimately, the emphasis that emerges is one on communities. Like other reports that would follow, 'Alarma' delineates a unified homosexual community (that never existed in this imagined way, neither in theory nor in practice) from its straight counterpart. Such a move presents the homosexual and the heterosexual as polar opposites (promiscuity versus monogamy, unclean gay sex versus clean heterosexual sex, urban vice versus traditional values and virtue) and establishes the vulnerability of the first over the immunity of the latter. The report even pays lip service to this fact when it notes that 'colectivos como el Frente de Liberación Homosexual de Andalucía han protestado públicamente, alegando que este tipo de noticias lesiona su imagen, ya que asegura [que] no existe ninguna enfermedad infecciosa exclusiva de los homosexuales' [groups such as the Homosexual Liberation Front of Andalucía have protested publicly, alleging that these types of reports harm their image, as they assure that no infectious disease exclusive to homosexuals exists]. Yet such protests are hardly relevant when the Spanish outbreak narrative has already been demonstratively established, when 'facts' can be supplied to separate those who are HIV-positive from those who are not, will not be, or who purportedly never could be.

In this manner, 'Alarma' could dismiss the protests of gay groups in Spain as the outcry of a community with a lot of bad baggage. The perceived ties between gays in Spain and gays in New York, San Francisco, or Los Angeles reaffirms the belief that all are equally tainted, whether socially, morally, or physically; the spread of 'their' illness to hemophiliacs, meanwhile, seems proof positive of the contagiousness of American decadence by way of African poverty. 'Alarma' concludes this section with a warning to its audience, who are imagined not to form part of these at-risk communities:

> Sea o no sea esta la etiología de la enfermedad, de ninguna manera presupone que aquellas personas que la pueden contraer a través del vehículo de la transfusión del plasma tengan nada que ver con la homosexualidad. Es necesaria la aclaración porque se han producido lamentables confusiones.[11]

One wonders what 'lamentable confusions' had occurred from the mere suggestion of homosexuality among hemophiliacs afflicted with

11 'Whether this is or is not the etiology of the illness, in no way does it mean that those who contract it through plasma transfusions have anything to do with homosexuality. This clarification is necessary, as there have been lamentable confusions.'

AIDS. Were the hemophiliacs treated as gay persons with AIDS? Was the care, compassion, or medical treatment they received made any less by their speculated association with a gay illness? And what really makes this lamentable: their treatment, or the fact that the hemophiliacs were not gay and were treated as such? Revealing a disdain for its homosexual populace—the believed originators of this sickness—belies the narrative of modernity and sexual freedoms that is so often attributed to the Spanish transition to democracy.

The remainder of 'Alarma' aims to fight against 'esta ceremonia de la confusión científica' [this ceremony of scientific confusion], a fairly stylized description of the uncertainty surrounding the origins of AIDS that nevertheless demonstrates the report's commitment to misunderstanding the global spread of the virus. That is, the confusion is not particularly scientific in nature. There was indeed a dearth of information available to the general populace at the outset, but this was compounded heavily by outside fears and prejudices, as we have seen in this very report. If, as Ed Cohen writes, 'conflicts about medical truths conceal conflicts of *values*' (2009, 275), we see the clearest of values being portrayed by the writers of the 'Alarma' report. Their resulting confusion, to that end, is one of strict moral values: that the illness refused to be relegated so neatly to homosexuals, that it continued to spread to other groups, and that the social and moral lines drawn as its borders seemed to constantly shift. New groups and peoples, in fact, were increasingly revealed to be vulnerable to AIDS, disrupting the sense of immunity established in its early years.

The brand of immunity outlined in these years, in some ways, is still in effect. That is, the nature of establishing at-risk groups meant that most groups were 'naturally' not at risk, that they were protected from AIDS by communal connections that might be spiritual, moral, geographical, or even racial. For that reason, to understand AIDS at this time in Spain as an issue of communities is to understand their relevance to contemporary Western constructions of illness itself. In *A Body Worth Defending: Immunity, Biopolitics, and the Apotheosis of the Modern Body*, Ed Cohen argues that modern perceptions of sickness and immunity are fully wrapped up in the political construction of community. Cohen writes that the legal concept of immunity in Rome and the political concept of self-defense described by figures such as Hobbes, both existing first as separate and distinct ideas, became fused together as 'biological immunity' around the late nineteenth century (2009, 3). The end result is a biopolitical concept that

> grafts or inoculates both military and political potentials into human biology as an entangled mode of explanation. In fact, immunity offers

> a peculiar hybrid of military, political, and biological thinking that 'naturally' negates the distinctions among these realms. Rendering biological immunity as an organism's active process of defense, scientific medicine deftly fuses a bellicose ideology (which sees environmental challenge as a hostile attack) with a political notion of legal exception (which nevertheless affirms the law's universal applicability). (2009, 6)

In other words, in separating the human organism as a frontier that must be defended, the body is both exposed and opposed to the others who would seek to negate its existence (Cohen 2009, 278). Thus, it is through biological immunity that the body becomes a discrete, defensible self that clearly distinguishes between the interior and the exterior, the domestic and the foreign, the self and the other. The political notions that come to buttress biological immunity, meanwhile, contribute to the sense of the self as a political concept, and envelop immunity in a complex interlocking of the political and the legal. The ensuing metaphors embroiled in such a distinction create hostile terrorists out of germs, cinematic villains out of index cases, and heroic narratives out of survivors.

The clash between biological immunity's interiorized construction of the self and the outsider also delineates and restricts the functions of modern medicine. Margaret Lock has noted how 'efforts to reduce suffering have habitually focused on the control and repair of individual bodies' (qtd in Cohen 2009, 272). Consequently, the outside realm of the social—as distinguished from the self's biological immunity—is disregarded: 'The social origins of suffering and distress, including poverty and discrimination, even if fleetingly recognized, are set aside, while effort is expended in controlling disease and averting death through biomedical manipulations' (qtd in Cohen 2009, 272). The unconcerned response of 'Alarma' to the outcries of gay groups in Spain, then, reveals the low social perception of gays, yes; however, it also underscores the perceived irrelevance of exterior social concerns (like discrimination) to the interior workings of biomedicine. Discrimination against a minority/outside group is of little importance to the larger sociopolitical community, then, which must defend its borders from attack.

The claims of 'scientific confusion' from 'Alarma', in this light, condemn the circulation of the outside into the interior realm of the biomedical. The report's insistence on separate, at-risk communities is a further way of marking these outside/inside narratives by establishing immunity for certain groups, and a contagious sort of vulnerability for others which must be continually defended against. The end result is a confusing metaphor, indeed, and postulates an interiorized body of the state that perceives the exterior threat of these communities as attacks on its discrete self. The struggle to understand the encroaching AIDS epidemic, and the war against the illness, 'paradoxically marshals, and indeed radically expands, the resources of immune discourse against an infectious agent which lays waste to the very defensive capabilities ascribed to immunity itself' (Cohen 2009, 278). Casting the body of the individual as a unit returns to the metaphor of the Hobbesian state itself, the body politic; the attack of AIDS on the body politic of Spain, in turn, has coded certain communities as germs intent on bringing the country to its knees.

In 'Alarma', the focus on the hemophiliac brothers and on hemophilia itself is a way of demonstrating the outsider threat that AIDS represents to the Spanish public, an attestable link between a foreign illness and domestic death. In a similar fashion, 'SIDA: La enfermedad de los 80' aims to showcase the impact of homosexuals in the AIDS crisis while quarantining the main effects of the illness to the United States. First aired on August 20, 1983 (only three months after 'Alarma'), 'La enfermedad de los 80' was the second report with an exclusive focus on the AIDS epidemic to be broadcast on RTVE. Like 'Alarma', its images of the 'gay plague' revert to familiar homosexual stereotypes while reifying an increasingly blatant Spanish outbreak narrative within its hemophiliac community; unlike 'Alarma', however, the full focus on the United States seems designed to temper public fears in Spain about the reach of the epidemic. If AIDS could be demonstrated as belonging to this outsider community, it might shore up the defensible borders of the Spanish body politic.

'La enfermedad de los 80' opens inauspiciously enough, with a familiar tale of AIDS run rampant among homosexuals and an assortment of 'facts' that are meant to explain the illness:

> Cada año los homosexuales reivindican sus derechos con desfiles por las principales ciudades de EE. UU. Este año, las manifestaciones son diferentes. Una enfermedad conocida como 'SIDA' se ha extendido por toda la comunidad gay... Hasta la fecha, en un 70% de los casos de SIDA, han estado implicados homosexuales. No es raro, pues, que el SIDA haya sido apodado rápidamente como 'la peste de los gay'. ('SIDA: La enfermedad de los 80' 1983)[12]

12 'Each year, homosexuals claim their rights through marches throughout the main cities of the United States. This year, the protests are different. An illness known as "AIDS" has spread throughout the gay community... To date, 70% of AIDS cases have involved homosexuals. It is not surprising, therefore, that AIDS has been quickly dubbed "the gay plague".'

As it describes homosexual protests and panic in the face of the gay scourge of AIDS, the report cycles through a selection of images that combine frivolity and activism in curious ways. Initial shots of homosexual pride parades demonstrate a color guard, men performing choreographed movements in a parade march, others who dance and carry flags, others dressed in leather and enjoying themselves. The celebratory images slowly begin to focus in on certain details: men wearing armbands with AIDS in an interdictory circle and banners that decry the spread of AIDS set amid the images of celebrations, for example. The mixture of AIDS activism with the celebration of a pride parade seems designed to suggest an unconcerned, casual viewpoint toward the extension of AIDS threaded around the purported decadence of the homosexual community. The figures provided by the report, meanwhile, relegate AIDS to a homosexual illness, and find it 'unsurprising' that AIDS should be known as the gay plague. The result, in just the first minute of the report, is a heavily loaded mixture that blames the gay community's hedonism and shames its response to AIDS as insufficient.

The report continues by noting how AIDS 'ha atacado' [has attacked] major cities in the United States before declaring that 'existe una histeria generalizada en los EEUU' [a general hysteria exists in the United States]. As it goes forward, the report makes repeated reference to people with AIDS as 'victims' of the illness. While this sort of language is practically standard even today, its resorting to bellicose metaphors of illness demonstrates how illness is a perceived threat to biological immunity and the defensible borders of the body politic of the larger community/state. This is to say that bestowing AIDS with the sentience of an attacking agent marks it as enemy, which in turn loads a 'putatively nonpolitical position' (Cohen 2009, 277) with a very real set of politics. Similar to the claim that one is just reporting the facts of the matter, the language of attack/victim constructs a specific scenario of the world, one in which the virus is an enemy combatant on the battlefield of the human body—and the victims are the fallen in battle. The language of attack/victim or friend/enemy, as Cohen notes, 'in no way derives from the matter of the world; it does not describe the unfolding of biochemical processes according to immutable natural laws; it does not constitute an unmediated representation of an essential physical truth' (2009, 277). The metaphors created in this type of language demonstrate how profoundly political AIDS had become, even in these early years and even in what seems to be the smallest of verbal slippages.

The language of attacks, ills, and enemies also begins to separate the boundaries of an ill community from a healthy one. Centering on San Francisco as the epitome of one such ill community, 'La enfermedad de los

80' moves from citywide panoramas to its bustling streets, with images that bubble with sexuality. In a short sequence, two men face the camera as a third shirtless man walks toward them in passing. The man in the center of the image slowly and admiringly follows the shirtless man with his gaze, turning his head and watching him as he walks by. Another brief sequence shows a tight close-up on a man wearing nothing but bright red shorts; the camera follows his brisk, shimmying walk for a few seconds. As these images flash on screen, the report notes ominously:

> Esta enfermedad es de difícil diagnóstico. Tarda en manifestarse. Puede que muchos de los que estén afectados por ella aún no lo sepan [13]... No se conoce cura alguna para esta dolencia. Nadie sabe exactamente cómo se contrae ni cómo se contagia.

But these words ring hollow against the veritable parade of gay male sexuality on display, in the glistening male bodies that walk across the screen. Even as the report laments that no one knows how AIDS is spread or contracted, the camera focuses tightly on the image of the man's ass in motion. What does this suggest except a suspicion and fear of gay male sexuality? Perhaps no one truly knew what brought about AIDS, but 'La enfermedad de los 80' makes a direct correlation between the emergence of the illness and the flagrant sexuality of gay men in the United States in ways that are obvious and concerted.

In theory, constructing the outbreak narrative in this manner allowed Spanish media to articulate Spain's ideological difference from its American neighbors as well as demonstrate the safety of its healthy and non-tainted community of citizens. This was a flawed strategy, clearly, as the rising number of AIDS cases in Spain almost immediately belied any suggestion of immunity within its borders. For this reason, both this report and 'Alarma' had to establish risk groups that could be considered separate and divisible from the larger body politic. As Wald writes, 'the balance of the community marked by immunity is always precarious, with the requisite number of strangers ... weighing constantly against the threat of too many strangers, hence social breakdown or anarchy in politics and germs' (2008, 57). We should consider how both of these RTVE reports structure their narratives along the lines of the stranger, who alternately becomes a homosexual, a hemophiliac, or an intravenous drug user. If biological immunity requires that we think of the self in terms of a bordered entity that is both exposed

13 'This disease is difficult to diagnose. It takes time to manifest. Many of those who may be affected by it still do not know it ... There is no known cure for this ailment. No one knows exactly how it is contracted nor how it is spread.'

and attacked—and if the same holds true when immunity is grafted back into the metaphor of the body politic—then establishing the 'stranger' or the 'outside' (in Cohen's terminology) is a way of identifying the dangerous element that threatens our borders.

Wald's reminder that the stranger/outsider is also part and parcel of how we define the boundaries between community and other is equally important, particularly given the common historical practices of quarantine and exile in illness. When the stranger (whether it be AIDS, the threat of homosexuality, or a globalizing populace influenced by foreign cultures) has already invaded the borders of the body politic, something like a political 'autoimmune response' occurs that identifies risk groups, separates them from the community-at-large, and casts aspersions on their identifiable characteristics as different and dangerous from the dominant culture. As critics such as Smith or de Miguel and Kirp have shown, such a move went against the theoretically liberated ideology of Spanish democracy; but as has also been noted, Spanish political ideology was never so fully liberated as the discourse of the times suggested. Regardless, whatever positive characteristics the stranger may have provided—multiculturalism, increased diversity of sexual practices and politics, a theoretically more democratic environment—were shuffled off in favor of an outbreak narrative that reduced specific differences to inherent threats to community health and the wellbeing of the state.

As 'La enfermedad de los 80' documents the move from gay panic to generalized AIDS panic (and eventually back again), it notes how heterosexuals have also been affected by AIDS, particularly hemophiliacs and drug users. In a remarkably similar cluster of images, the report details each group and their specific risk of AIDS infection. Describing hemophiliacs as 'propensos a sangrar abundantemente por la más mínima herida' [prone to bleeding profusely from the slightest wound], the report explains the necessity of blood coagulant as a lifesaving tool for them. Since this coagulant is extracted from donor blood, 'muchos científicos afirman que éste es el agente transmisor' [many scientists claim that this is the transmitting agent]. The voiceover that sketches hemophilia in these broad terms continues, as a (presumably hemophiliac) man is showing giving himself an injection. This sequence immediately cuts to a description of intravenous drug users, who are 'el segundo mayor grupo y representan el 16% de todos los casos' [the second largest group, accounting for 16% of all cases].[14] While relaying this information on drug usage, a young man is

14 Although the report does not make this explicit, the claim that drug users represented 16% of all users seems to rely on the global data available at the time

shown injecting himself. Like the hemophiliac the report has just shown, the man occupies the center of the frame, his arm tied off and the needle just entering his arm. Both sequences follow the same loose progression of shots: a close-up shot focuses on the man's face, head bent and intently focused on what he is doing; a second close-up on the point of insertion in the arm; finally, a switch to a medium shot that shows the man from waist up with his arm extended, hand balled into a fist, and inserting the needle. The visual similarities between the sequences of the hemophiliac and the drug user are striking, and their coupling in this report suggests a loose, thematic correlation between the two as dependent on a chemical substance that can both prolong and destroy lives. As with the images of the homosexual community earlier, a person is reduced to a risky, poorly understood practice that endangers life.

All the same, and despite the correlation between the three risk groups, the type of practice still matters. Is the practice a sexual act linked to drugs, lurid bars, and perceived as filthy? Is it a damning need for an addictive drug, seen as a consequence of bad behavior or poor willpower? Or is it a lifesaving drug necessitated by a faulty body? Even while casually looping the three groups together, 'La enfermedad de los 80' makes clear the difference of the hemophiliac. He appears to be middle-aged, dressed in a shirt and tie and is seated on a couch in a living room. Behind him is a window, with a view to a yard lush with vegetation. On the table before him and to his side are the materials he needs for his injection of blood coagulant. The *mise en scène* evokes family life, relative wealth, health, and class. The drug user, in contrast, is younger, dressed more casually, and has a visible tattoo on his forearm. He sits in a windowless, sterile environment that is reminiscent of a hospital or a jail cell. There is no window to the outside in this tiled, white room. His age links him to the rising drug culture among youth in Spain, and his location institutionalizes the illicitness of his act into an authoritative system of medical and judicial power. Although these men are presented as little more than their risky practices, the hemophiliac alone is linked to the theoretically stable, wholesome, and private space of the home; the lawlessness of the drug user is contained within systems of power, and the homosexuals are public displays of unhealthy sex.

As in 'Alarma', this works to define AIDS as a very particular type of illness that affects a small group of preselected communities. These communities are in turn defined by and made beholden to the inherently

rather than data specific to Spain. As discussed in the Introduction and in Chapter 4, it has been shown that, despite the index cases touted in the Spanish media, HIV/AIDS was largely spread through intravenous drug transmission in Spain.

risky practices they perform, practices that expose them to the virus that causes AIDS. Structuring the illness as a disease that follows strict lines of community and immunity, these reports reify the outbreak narrative that defines innocent victims and deliberate, willful transgressors. Spain and the Spanish people—who are categorized in the majority as normal, and as such outside these risk groups—are to watch from the sidelines as this illness unfolds and runs through these communities. Unlike 'Alarma', however, 'La enfermedad de los 80' refrains from africanizing the illness, a move that is in sharp contrast with the general tendency to collapse Africa and Haiti into each other as primordial cradles of death. Instead, it places the blame for the 'mystery' of AIDS, as it refers to the virus's origins, at the pedicured feet of the well-traveled homosexual community: 'El por qué los haitianos son víctimas del SIDA nadie lo sabe realmente. Una posible explicación puede ser que Haití es uno de los lugares favoritos de vacaciones de los homosexuales americanos. Posiblemente trajeron consigo la enfermedad desde América' [No one really knows why Haitians are victims of AIDS. One possible explanation may be that Haiti is a favorite vacation spot among gay Americans. Perhaps they brought the disease with them from America] ('SIDA: La enfermedad de los 80' 1983). In another move that betrays the structuring of its own outbreak narrative, the report quickly follows with figures of Haitians with AIDS—it notes that 35 Haitian immigrants to the US reportedly had HIV, while there were 50 cases on the island itself—a move which attempts to juxtapose scientific reporting with its suppositional evidence. The spread of AIDS is thus linked to economic, cultural, and sexual decadence, and the mobility of the homosexual is placed alongside his flagrant displays of sexuality and skin, willfully and dangerously spreading its illness.

The closing images in the report cement this vision further. After running through the primary groups at risk and demonstrating the scant need for worry among the general Spanish public, the report returns to the spread of AIDS among homosexuals. As it describes a (non-specified) American-based foundation that helps gay people living with AIDS, displaying pamphlets for the prevention of the illness, the report concludes: 'Muchos homosexuales piensan que no se está haciendo lo suficiente para ayudarles, aunque se estén gastando varios millones de dólares en investigaciones. Se sienten más discriminados que nunca a consecuencia del SIDA' [Many homosexuals think that not enough is being done to help them, even though various millions of dollars are being spent on research. They feel more discriminated against than ever as a consequence of AIDS.] The information, while more or less true, hinges on its 'aunque' [even though], which asserts that an unknown but vast quantity of money is being spent on homosexuals, undermining their claims that not enough is being done. Additionally, the clips displayed at this moment show men and women sunbathing in a park. The contrast is at once highly ironic and biting: it suggests laziness and an almost regal decadence in the homosexual community amid the turmoil caused by their risky behaviors. 'La enfermedad de los 80' is bookended by the gay body's prowling sexuality and its spoiled luxuriance; it is a stranger's body on display, dangerous, greedy, and infectious. The insidious nature of the virus hidden in this body, meanwhile, lends these images a predatory sheen.

It should be clear that both 'Alarma' and 'La enfermedad de los 80' were theoretically impartial and apolitical reports that nevertheless demonstrate the full weight of a media machine bent on constructing an outbreak narrative for Spain. The Spanish index cases that appeared and reappeared (the anonymous gay man in 1982 and the hemophiliac children in 1983) corroborated a global story that defined particular risk groups and the risky practices that they undertook. Initially delineating these groups either as tainted by foreign influence—global homosexual culture, the globalized drug trafficking industry, American donors of blood coagulant—or as inherently foreign themselves, the Spanish outbreak narrative soon adjusted itself to drawing clear distinctions between a dominant, traditional Spanish culture and these risk groups. The resulting narrative followed an organizational structure categorized by close adherence to the matched concepts of biological immunity and political community, wherein the attacking virus was physical, cultural, and social. The theoretically closed 'risk groups' left in the wake of the first years of AIDS were bracketed, marked as outside the borders of what constituted the truly Spanish. If the state is an 'immunological ecosystem', to crib from Wald, and 'the health and safety of the citizens is linked to national borders' (2008, 57), these reports demonstrate the ways that Spanish media began to shore up complex notions of statehood and cultural life through illness and AIDS.

What happens to the real people who are affected by this illness—those who have been made into exemplary risk groups, those who perished and became representations of a bad set of bad practices? The insistence on the index case betrays a blinding need for a singular truth in the murkiness of illness. We want to know and understand an illness, even when that knowledge may be simply a sum of cobbled-together facts: a geographical location, a person-cum-index case, and a date or moment that can be captured and examined. There is a difference between a truth and its meaning, or between data and the narratives that both cloud and control it.

The reliance on an index case, on the truth of a medical narrative coupled with a mythology of healthy community, dangerously collapses our experience of life and illness. The origin story trusses up our affective relationship to illnesses with medical science. We can point to a man in 1981 who contracted HIV on a trip, read the SIDA STUDI graph that finds cases in the 1950s on the African continent, hear the news reports of the hemophiliac brothers—but these are stories, index cases that have been mixed and remixed freely with fiction, journalism, and medicine. We know that AIDS happened—still happens—in Spain because of its effects; the ascription of meaning to anything else betrays our fears of illness, contagion, and getting and staying sick.

CHAPTER TWO

Bad Blood

In its early stages—and in the most cynical and cruel of interpretations—AIDS was perceived as an illness through which one got what one deserved. The infection and deaths of homosexuals and intravenous drug users, the viral spread through prison populations and networked clusters of friends and lovers, and the nebulous sense of something dire occurring in the United States all reinforced Spanish public opinion of AIDS as somebody else's monstrous problem. As discussed in Chapter 1, Spanish news reports, newspaper articles, films, and television sought to quell the potential of rising panic by reminding their audiences that the threat to the public at large was minimal. As time passed and the disease spread, however, and as new swaths of the population were revealed to be vulnerable and exposed, the steadfast belief in one's righteous impermeability to AIDS was put under pressure. Who could be protected from this virus, if it could be everywhere, and how could one possibly shelter from it?

In the face of increasing vulnerability and susceptibility to the taint of illness—which was never only physical, but also social and cultural—a narrative pattern began to emerge in these early years that framed AIDS along familiar, Manichean lines, relegating its diffused presence to cleanly divided categories: purity and pollution. In this narrative, victimhood was a status that one had to earn, not a natural state of physical precarity, and HIV/AIDS was a dark presence that lurked hidden in the body. One's susceptibility to the virus was measured in powerfully moralizing ways, and the true victim was ultimately seen to be a wild amalgam of conundrums: healthy but infected, innocent but tainted, and marginal to the depravity of AIDS while remaining central to the purported normalcy of the nation. This resignification appropriated purity and cleanliness from those theoretically less deserving of its status (read: the guilty, those who brought the illness upon themselves) to more fully care for the political, social, and figural representations of the future of the nation and its normative institutions. Such a move, as we will see, came from sources such as national associations, print and media outlets, health agencies, and local and national governmental institutions, to name a few. Together, they emphasized national ideals of healthy childhoods and sturdy family structures while working to remove tainted risk groups, unhealthy bodies, and dangerous citizens from their midst.

The push to protect 'the child' (as emblematic of all children, of childhood, and of the normative family) was a way to protect some sense of a future for Spain, even as its young democracy struggled to find its footing in the global arena and even as the 'blood crisis' that erupted in these years further strengthened the threat to national futures. Panic surged as the future, that place of limitless possibility and hope that is so often embodied in the next generation, was placed under attack by an enigmatic virus that seemed to spring from nowhere; for that reason, and as the narratives clustering around AIDS in its early years coalesced into stories of dangerous practices, the figure of the child became the exemplary victim, an innocent who had been placed in harm's way. Blood, in this same period, was made into a boogeyman of monumental proportions, a conduit for fears of impurity, deviance, and reprobate sexuality. This figural child was not to blame for contracting an illness, neither adherent to risky practices nor guilty of sexual misconduct, and thus became emblematic of a normative Spanish society: straight, pure, and now susceptible to a disease that it seemingly had no hand in bringing about.

In Chapter 1, I discussed the origin stories that were created from the AIDS index cases in Spain, and how they presented specific risky groups and actions as threatening. The reports on Juan Antonio and Diego de los Reyes Mesa, the hemophiliac brothers who died in 1983 after receiving tainted blood product, sensationally highlighted the brothers' innocence and blamelessness as dissimilar to the spread of HIV/AIDS in other countries and as symbolic of a sort of social reckoning: the sins of the present laying waste to the presumed innocence of the future. Regardless of the truth of this, the act of marking these two as index cases of AIDS (the first to fall to the disease, the cases around which the story of AIDS in Spain could be constructed) shaped the nascent discourse surrounding the illness in a variety of ways: it underscored the very serious problem that hemophiliacs were only just beginning to face, it cast a spotlight on the ever-important figure of the child, the normative repository of the future (Edelman 2004), it contributed to blood debates and the proliferation of blood metaphors, and it further tied the democratic politics of Spain to the health of its body politic.

The deaths of these two brothers became a story, a plot point in the early narratives of what AIDS could and did mean in Spain. But in some ways, the child is always a story that we tell ourselves. That is, and following Kathryn Bond Stockton in *The Queer Child, or Growing Sideways in the Twentieth Century* (2009), we create our narratives of childhood in hindsight, always from the vantage point of adulthood and looking backwards into the foggy glass of memory. In that manner, childhood can be co-opted and reconfigured as a state of being with deep meaning for future societies. In the types of narratives that crop up around illness, childhood is particularly significant: it is a symbol, a means to project fears of uninhibited sexuality and mortality onto a figure representative of purity and futurity. The figure of the child, then, is often made to collude with a narrative that fits a normative future. That future, in turn, ensures continuity on a broad level—genetic, social, and cultural. When childhood is utilized in this manner, it is as a promise that the world as we know it will continue. Illness, among many other things, complicates this promise.

But as we shall see, children can be chaotic, unruly, and can refuse the paths that have been laid before them. The figure of the child, that creature that appears in the stories and reports and mediated representations in this chapter, may likewise reject or fall short of the narratives into which we have placed it. This is to say that childhood is also a lived experience—whether we fail to fully capture it in our adult recollection is another matter. The reality foregrounding these popular notions of childhood-as-symbolic-innocence is full of very real children, mundanely literal kids; and we cannot forget, within the sensationalistic reports that utilized children as props and symbols to make a larger political and social point, that there actually were children dying during the outbreak of AIDS in Spain. In pointing out just how the symbolic figure of the child has been used propagandistically in these AIDS narratives, it seems easy to forget the children themselves, which is a different sort of dangerous narrative to promote. This chapter's careful separation of the way the child 'functioned' symbolically and literally (or imagistically and medically) during the early years of AIDS in Spain is, in some ways, an attempt to allay the casual erasure of actual childhood. In learning more of what the figure of the child with AIDS meant, there will most certainly be something to learn about our sustained connections to childhood, youth, mortality, our blood, and ourselves.

There is a careful balancing act to be maintained, then: not to collude entirely with the nostalgia that seeks to protect childhood as a bastion of innocence and futurity, but neither to let go of childhood's symbolic import in everything from politics to media to cultural products. The early news reports, articles, and television specials that were disseminated in the period from 1981 to 1987 in Spain latched onto the figure of the child and its marred purity in the face of the increasingly monstrous virus. This chapter takes a selection of these for close analysis, particularly a few of the televised news reports from RTVE in this period, which frequently revert to images of infected children and childhood. The first broadcast on AIDS from RTVE, 'Alarma: El virus que viene de California' (May 14, 1983), was discussed in Chapter 1 but has renewed importance here. In fact, of the other twenty-something special broadcasts on AIDS on RTVE from 1983 to 1987, nearly half make direct reference to children and childhood in a variety of ways.[1] As we will see in this chapter, when coupled with the blood crisis that surrounded the illness in the 1980s, the fear of AIDS infection in minors took a frenzied tone.

This is not to say that such a tone was unwarranted, or not without its own rationale. The numbers for HIV/AIDS infection are notoriously slippery (and any belief in the 'truth' of such figures must be continually checked against the awareness of who provides them and to what end), and attempting to lay them out encourages pathologization and a problematic adherence to the risk groups defined in the illness's first years. Despite this assertion, it seems clear that the most frightening of these early figures belonged to hemophiliacs, whose infection rate spiked dramatically between 1981 and 1985. Although this will be underscored later in this chapter, it is worth noting that in 1982, as the reports of AIDS began to emerge in Spain, there were upwards of 2,000 known hemophiliac patients. In 1985, with the advent of new procedures that limited the Spanish hemophiliac community's reliance on foreign blood supplies and provided for a more stringent purification process of the coagulant used in treating hemophilia, HIV/AIDS infection rates for hemophiliacs had practically reached a standstill. According to the coordinator of the Hemophiliac Center in Madrid's La Paz Hospital, by this period there were some 1,100 hemophiliacs infected with HIV/AIDS, an infection rate above 50% of its known population in Spain (Federación Española de Hemofilia 1993, 9).[2]

1 The following list is just a sampling of the news reports that dealt in some substantial way with childhood and youth in this time period: 'SIDA: Crece la alarma' [AIDS: The Growing Alarm], September 15, 1985; *Más vale prevenir*, June 16, 1985, and January 9, 1987; *Generación 800*, September 19, 1985; *El domingo es nuestro*, March 15, 1987; 'La enfermedad y el miedo' [Sickness and Fear], April 23, 1987; and 'Incidencia del SIDA en la población escolar infantil' [Incidence of AIDS among Schoolchildren], August 13, 1987.

2 Astonishingly, this seems by most accounts to be a fairly conservative estimate. An issue of *Fedhemo* estimated the infection percentage at 60–70% of Spain's hemophiliacs (Tusell 1993, 17), while the *Canadian Medical Association Journal* wrote that '82% of [Spain's] 2700 hemophiliacs were infected with HIV' due to its reliance on blood-clotting products from the United States (Dunn 1993, 612).

These devastating numbers would mark the hemophiliac community in Spain for decades to come, but the damage would also reach further out, as the creeping spread of this so-called mysterious illness into Spanish bodies disturbed the inherent symbolism of blood as life giving and life sustaining and disrupted a sense of national and racial identity. If your very blood works against you, threatens you, and makes you sick, what happens to your hopes of life and vitality? To take that a step further: what happens to the national hopes of vitality and prosperity in this moment, with the specter of polluted blood looming large?

The unified fictions that promise futurity, purity, and national identity in the symbolic import ascribed to both children and blood saw themselves increasingly threatened by an illness that refused to stay relegated to theoretically fringe social groups. As more and more hemophiliacs and children began to get sick, the notion of the child as symbolic of continuity writ large saw itself imperiled, sexualized, and associated with a frightening and life-altering illness. AIDS tainted the perception of the blood's purity and altered the promise of the future, and it became increasingly difficult to discuss AIDS without conjuring sexuality, mortality, and monstrosity in the same breath. The havoc that the illness wrought, in this manner, was more than just physical. What kind of lasting effect might it have when the lens through which one imagines future iterations of society is itself cracked, darkened, or shattered completely? By recoding the symbolic nature of childhood and the normative family unit, the narratives attributed to AIDS inserted mortality into a story that had been filled with utopian, democratic promise.

This chapter analyzes those bloody narratives, examining how the disease mutated and reworked existing ideas of childhood and sanguinary purity through concepts of victimhood and guilt. I also claim that HIV/AIDS provided a means of queering these metaphors and figures, even when it seemed to reify their place within the promises of democracy. In the first half of this chapter, I note the emphasis placed on childhood and children in the stories of HIV-positive hemophiliacs, and how these stories shaped the larger narrative of AIDS in Spain even as they were crafted to isolate the disease from the public at large; in the context of the ongoing blood debates of this period, these narratives reveal not only their urgency but their ongoing impact in cultural understandings of who belongs within the national body and who does not. The second half of the chapter turns to the figure of the hemophiliac, taking into account the visual language that is brought to bear in order to sanitize their image; here I examine journals, images, and articles that seek to cleanse the social threat of AIDS and promote the recuperation of the hemophiliac back within the boundaries of the risk-averse, even as the physical threat of AIDS was bearing down on all sides. Tying the polluted to the pure and the apocalyptic to the futurist, I see blood as a symbol of democratic promise and the fear of its failure. The end result of this moment in time converted the promise of generational futurity into the viral potential of HIV/AIDS, disrupting normalcy and national identity with the infectious spread of illness.

Infecting the family

Many of the texts, films, and assorted mediated representations of the child with AIDS that are studied in this chapter operate from the shared assumption that they know precisely who and what a child is, along with how to define and identify childhood. Perhaps it seems easy enough: one simply has to point to a human being who is 10 years old or younger, and we have identified a child. But the question, clearly, runs deeper. Paraphrasing the 'field-defining questions' made by Philippe Ariès in *Centuries of Childhood* (1962), Kathryn Bond Stockton defies such simplicity, inquiring: 'What makes a child? What conditions are needed historically for there to be creatures who are called "children"?' (2009, 40).[3] Indeed, and as I have briefly suggested above, modern configurations of these concepts rely on a set of shared beliefs and universalizations about everything from proper levels of innocence and sexuality to acceptable behaviors, age limits, dress codes, and appropriate intergenerational relationships. I make no claim to answer such questions or fully explore these concepts to any satisfactory degree in this chapter, but I do hope to disrupt the sense that childhood was a fully comprehended phenomenon for the directors, reporters, and audiences of the early reports and media on AIDS in Spain, reports that so often assumed a shared knowledge of and range of beliefs regarding childhood. By uncritically accepting common notions of children and childhood to be the only worthwhile definitions available to us, they are allowed to reflect back a vision of the world as we wish it to be constructed.

If childhood is always a distant past created from memory and recollection, a projection of our vaguely sensed past selves, then our representations of

3 As suggested here, Stockton is by no means the first to reconfigure Ariès' line of questioning, and indeed a whole area of studies has grown up around his *Centuries of Childhood*. It is beyond the scope of this book to attend in any profound way to the rich field of children's studies; for a more in-depth outline of the shape of its borders and the scope of its questions as pertaining to Spain, see *The Child in Spanish Cinema* (Wright 2013), *The Two cines con niño: Genre and the Child Protagonist in Fifty Years of Spanish Film (1955–2010)* (Hogan 2018), and *Inhabiting the In-Between: Childhood and Cinema in Spain's Long Transition* (Thomas 2019).

childhood can serve to explain key aspects of our social and affective lives. That is, the ways we imagine our lives to be (and to have been, as children) reveal some of the tropes that our very existences depend on; particularly, and most relevant to this chapter, we upend the fictions of health and innocence that are so often tied to the memory of youth and childhood. Our recreations and remembrances of children, following Stockton, both feed and demonstrate the 'queerness' of childhood.[4] She writes: 'The silences surrounding the queerness of children happen to be broken—loquaciously broken and broken almost only—by fictional forms. Fictions literally offer the forms that certain brooding on children might take' (2009, 2). We might understand the 'fictions' that Stockton writes about to be likewise tied to the persistent representations of childhood in the early news reports on AIDS, so reiterated and codified as to create their own sort of fabricated discourse. Saving the lives of children was indeed a concern for many in these early years, but what seems to be truly at work in these reports is an insistence that society itself be saved through the rescue and rehabilitation of children—and with it, Spain's future, promise, and potential.

Childhood, as intimated in the introduction to this chapter, thus operates principally (but not uniquely) around issues of perception. As Stockton writes, 'the child is precisely who we are and we are not and, in fact, never were. It is the act of adults looking back. It is a ghostly, unreachable fancy' (2009, 5). Borrowing from Karen Lury's work on the child in cinema, Sarah Wright similarly notes how 'constructions of the child or the child's experience are so often "a form of anthropomorphism" in the sense that they reveal adult investments in the child' (2013, 1). Our investments in the continuity of the future—and here we can think in broad lines, in the continuity of futures that are at once personal, political, cultural, and genetic—are deeply embedded within our fantasies and recreations of childhood and children. Such reiterations, it should by now be clear, rarely have anything to do with actual, literal children themselves. By attaching ourselves to the seemingly inherent promise of the vaguely defined future, we reify the child-as-construct and, as Lee Edelman has brilliantly and polemically noted, invest ourselves in political stasis. In his *No Future*, Edelman writes that the 'figural child alone embodies the citizen as an ideal' (2004, 11) and that, unlike the 'ghostly fancy' of Stockton's imagistic child, our representations of childhood have a damning effect:

4 For Stockton, the queerness of childhood is primarily but no means exclusively limited to a child's sexual ambiguity or ambivalence. Indeed, her opening salvo makes clear the broad application of queerness to childhood: 'If you scratch a child, you will find a queer, in the sense of someone "gay" or just plain strange' (2009, 1).

> The social order exists to preserve for this universalized subject, this fantastic Child, a notional freedom more highly valued than the actuality of freedom itself, which might, after all, put at risk the Child to whom such a freedom falls due. Hence, whatever refuses this mandate by which our political institutions compel the collective reproduction of the Child must appear as a threat not only to the organization of a given social order but also, and far more ominously, to social order as such, insofar as it threatens the logic of futurism on which meaning always depends. (Edelman 2004, 11)

The 'logic of futurism', to crib from Edelman, is concerned with reaffirming structures which already exist in order to preserve them for the future—or more precisely, for the imagined child of the future. Sinisterly, then, our attachments to a figural child work to '*affirm* a structure, to *authenticate* social order, which it then intends to transmit to the future ... That Child remains the perpetual horizon of every acknowledged politics, the fantastic beneficiary of every political intervention' (Edelman 2004, 3). The question of 'what childhood really means' thus reveals itself to be neither simple nor wholly benign.

In this configuration, our perceptional fictions of what a child 'means' are directly related to the upholding of political and cultural structures that affirm life and futurity. So what does illness 'do' to this political fantasy? What ideas of generational continuity are disrupted or destroyed within this structure of feeling sick, and what new ideas might be brought about in this disruption? The final moments of 'SIDA: Crece la alarma' [AIDS: The Growing Alarm], which aired on RTVE on September 15, 1985, seem to sketch out a hesitant answer, remarkably demonstrating the adult fantasies that delineate childhood, our insistence on tracking innocence as commodity, and the potential of illness to both disrupt and reify these. As the father of Rafael Lledó Inzenga, a 19-year-old hemophiliac, reflects on his son's fatal contraction and development of the illness, he adamantly divides the essential innocence of youth from the adult terrain of suffering within disease. Believing himself to be 'protecting' his son from the malignancy of knowledge (represented here as future suffering and imminent mortality), the father instead conscripts himself to psychic suffering:

> Para mí, hay una diferencia radical—dramática—entre el hecho de que un enfermo que padece del SIDA lo sepa o no lo sepa. Si lo sabe, sus condiciones existenciales son verdaderamente horribles. La sociedad no se puede hacer una idea de lo que esto significa para la persona que es consciente que tiene esta enfermedad. En el caso de mi

> hijo, afortunadamente, él no lo sabía, lo cual es un cambio también profundísimo. Mi hijo no sufrió de esta enfermedad—murió de esta enfermedad, pero no sufrió de esta enfermedad. El enfermo que sepa que tiene esta enfermedad, si no recibe—en un entorno de cariño y humanidad—si no recibe ese afecto, desde luego es algo espantoso. La sociedad no sabe qué es esto. ('SIDA: Crece la alarma' 1985)[5]

In what can only be described as an attempt to protect the figural youth of his son—a youth also under physical attack from illness—the father fought to bear the psychic burden of AIDS so that his son would not have to. In this way, the report clearly identifies the stigmas associated with children with HIV/AIDS along with a dogged, adult insistence on the child's repeated purification. Youth must not be tainted nor overcome with the 'truly horrible existential conditions' of the person with AIDS, and the figure of the child must be continually recuperated, revivified, and its innocence reasserted.

Further detailing the conditions of his son's death and disease in an interview with *El País*, Rafael's father explains that his son 'nunca supo lo que padecía, nunca tuvo conciencia de que iba a morir. Siempre esperó sanar, hasta el final, hasta el último día, incluso hacía proyectos para las próximas vacaciones' [he never knew what he suffered from, he never knew that he was going to die. He always hoped to get better until the end, until the final day, even making plans for his next vacation] (Rivas 1985). Such fierce protection of Rafael's life raises questions about where childhood begins and ends—not in a developmental sense, but in a relational one. Rafael's age may not line up exactly with the usual notions of what childhood comprises, but the repeated emphasis on his need for protection—a safeguarding that must come at all costs—suggests that sustaining his innocence was a vital necessity that went beyond his own life. The opening of the article, for example, laments his youth as particularly tragic: 'Rafael Lledó Inzenga hubiese cumplido 20 años el primero de mayo si el SIDA no le hubiese matado exactamente dos meses antes' [Rafael Lledó Inzenga would have turned 20 on the first of May if AIDS hadn't killed him exactly two months previously] (Rivas 1985).

5 'For me, there is a radical difference—a dramatic one—between whether a patient who suffers from AIDS knows it or not. If he knows, his existential conditions are truly awful. Society has no idea what it means to the person who is aware of having this condition. In the case of my son, fortunately, he did not know, which is also a profound difference. My son did not suffer from this disease—he died of this disease, but he did not suffer from this disease. The patient who knows that he has this disease, if he does not receive—in an environment of care and humanity—if he does not receive that affection, it is certainly something awful. Society does not know what this is like.'

The choice of the verb 'matar', to kill, is intentionally aggressive, violently personifying the syndrome that the teen succumbed to as a brutal and chaotic murderer of an innocent.

In a manner that similarly correlates innocence to one's vital worth, Rafael's father speaks of his efforts to cordon off the blunt realities of HIV/AIDS in an attempt to block out its social impact and stigma. By his own account, he succeeded in doing so, avoiding what he deemed to be the indignities of the hospital: 'Eran inútiles los cuidados y el tratamiento, y el ingreso en un hospital presentaba dos aspectos negativos: que Rafa pudiese descubrir lo que padecía, y el aislamiento en que se encontraría allí. En casa vivía en su mundo. Su cuarto era su mundo' [The care and treatments were useless, and hospital admission had two negative aspects: that Rafa might discover what he was suffering from, and the isolation that would find there. At home, he lived in his world. His room was his world] (Rivas 1985). Confined to his room, which his father tellingly describes as his entire world, Rafael was cordoned off from the social stigma of HIV/AIDS. His father created a pure space of innocence, his childhood room, and encouraged him to hope and believe in the future. By sequestering him in this way, as his father sees it, Rafael's life and death were ultimately protected, and his innocence kept intact. But how could this space be so pure, or the teen so docilely led to his bed? Did he ask to go outside? Did he want to bring friends over, to go to school, to see a girl or a boy who he had a crush on? Was he only pure innocence, beaming at his father and making plans for the next day or week? In short, is it possible that Rafael was sustained only by the hope in tomorrow?

This is not to be read as wholesale condemnation of the father's actions, made in grief and out of what he believed to be the best for his family. It is, however, a demonstration of the ways that we shepherd childhood, how childhood is correlated with innocence, and how illness can thwart our attempts at promoting futurity through the child's cherubic likeness. The father chains himself to the knowledge of his son's imminent death and the physical ravages of disease so that his son might ostensibly be free from them, preventing the contamination of youth from mortality and suffering, and in so doing he protects general notions of unblemished childhood. But where is the real, actual son in this image? As his father finishes his statement in the RTVE special report, a sweet, light music plays over the interview, a sound not unlike that of a lullaby. Images of Rafael fill the screen: first as a baby, then as a young boy, before closing on a family portrait of happier times. No portrait of Rafael as a teenager, no image that might disturb this portrait of innocence. In this equation of youthfulness and happiness, suffering is the terrain of adults, not youth.

Along these lines, Stockton notes how we seek to safeguard at all costs 'the normative child—or the child ... on its path to normativity' (2009, 30). Something like this is at work here, for while the hemophiliac child is not precisely 'normal' in health (when normal is so often equated with the absence of sickness), the impulse to protect him or her from illness remains the same. Knowing that his son would succumb to opportunistic infections brought about by HIV, the father chose stasis over growth, correlating ignorance to innocence and thus needing his child to remain a child, essentially, forever—not only but especially in death. As Stockton writes, 'adults walk the line—the impossible line—of keeping the child at once what it is (what adults are not) and leading it toward what it cannot (at least, as itself) ever be (what adults are)' (2009, 30–31). Following Stockton's formulation, the thing that we as adults cannot ever be is, of course, the type of innocent, figural children that we have fabricated as symbols of futurity. Edelman's argument follows a similar tack, decrying the circular notions of futurity that animate political and public discourse and stating that 'we are no more able to conceive of a politics without a fantasy of the future than we are able to conceive of a future without the figure of the Child' (2004, 11).

The children that began to die in the early years of the AIDS epidemic in Spain drew attention to a multi-tiered problem that crossed political ideals, medical practices, and cultural beliefs. That is, the spread of the epidemic cut through the democratic promises of newness and futurity that the newly formed Spanish government drew its power and capital from, but it also unraveled the medical practices and procedures that had sustained the hemophiliac community and bit into the cultural beliefs that promoted what 'childhood' meant. The perceptions of childhood that activate daily life were broken down when facing AIDS and HIV, and the promise of a hopeful, democratic future was infected with perishability. Yet as we see from the father's protective shielding of his son, the infected child can also be used to sustain a normative sense of innocence and futurity, even from within the disturbing and subverting presence of illness.[6]

6 A note about my continued juxtaposition of the potential of illness to disturb figural childhood and its subsequent quashing in some of these texts: if the end result of the confluence of children and sickness is that our notions of childhood are kept in place, it could be asserted that illness simply reifies such constructs. My argument here is that the potential of illness to disturb, reconfigure, or 'queer' the notional child is constant, and that illness does in fact exercise a change in the construct of childhood that disturbs its forms and fantasies—despite the outcome of such a disturbance. To that end, I want to insist on its possibility and potential without always imagining that these are already lost from the outset.

In Chapter 1, I analyzed the 1983 report 'Alarma: El virus que viene de California' (May 14, 1983) as particularly important in crafting the outbreak narrative of AIDS in Spain. 'Alarma', as noted in that chapter, provided the first televised coverage of the AIDS epidemic in Spain, identifying the index cases of the illness as the Reyes Mesa brothers. It is worth revisiting this report briefly to see just how the figure of the child—and the actual bodies of children—informed the report, and how youth and futurity have always been wrapped into the conceptualizations of the illness in Spain. After briefly describing the foreign origins of the illness and tentatively assigning blame to gay men (particularly, those in San Francisco), the report spends its remaining time crafting an AIDS origin story that exclusively pertained to the hemophiliac children of Spain. In this version of the Spanish AIDS outbreak narrative, reporters visit the Virgen del Rocío Hospital in Sevilla, Spain, commenting that AIDS was first discovered in its transfusions wing.[7] A physician, Eduardo Lissen Otero, describes the discovery of what would eventually be known as HIV antibodies in the blood of the children, and the camera pans to show an image of children in hospital beds; as the report cuts back to the doctor and he continues his remarks, a child can be seen lying in bed next to him, calmly listening to the highly medical explanation. The subsequent scenes shift to a second doctor, Antonio Núñez, who describes what happens to the body and the immune system when these come into contact with the virus. As he begins speaking, he looks straight into the camera, directing his explanation to the television audience. He continues, and the program jumps throughout his explanation to shots of physicians visiting sick patients and bags of recently donated plasma. This parade of physicians continues as a third (José Manuel Jiménez Jiménez) and fourth doctor (Rafael Castro Artigas) explain the purportedly limited connotations of the outbreak of AIDS within hemophiliacs. This segment ends with the reporter interviewing a family with a hemophiliac child. The child is asked a barrage of questions about his treatment and care in the hospital, how he currently feels, and finally, what he wants to be when he grows up.

'Alarma: El virus que viene de California' has evident and at times commendable aims, particularly as the first televised report on AIDS in Spain: notably, it seeks to educate and pacify its viewers, assuaging their panic by giving a public face to the AIDS outbreak. The quiet, sick kids

7 As we have seen, this is not quite true to the complete timeline, and serves as another example of one of a few 'first encounters' of AIDS reported in Spain; notably, the anonymous gay man in the Vall d'Hebron hospital, and the intravenous drug user in the Hospital Clínic of Barcelona, two other origin narratives discussed in Chapters 1 and 4, respectively.

that populate this report, serenely gazing toward the camera from their hospital beds or being interviewed about their future goals and aspirations, are meant to demystify the illness's 'enigmatic' nature, limit its scope to a purportedly minuscule segment of the populace, and further belief in the irrepressible vigor of youth. How else might we understand the reporter who quizzes the sick child on his future, except as a portrayal of the future hope the child embodies, despite the assault of illness? Yet as laudable as these aims might be in theory, they are hardly innocuous. Tracking AIDS to an isolated outbreak within a small, medically controlled community, the report insists on the possibility of escaping the clutches of illness; by connecting the representation of the illness to images of children, it suggests resilience, optimism, and the potential to grow up and away from AIDS. The end result implies that there is a way to avoid this illness, that the viewer at home can be healthy, and that AIDS can be evaded. Reducing the reach of AIDS to a limited group (hemophiliacs) and funneling their representation through a barrage of images of children, 'Alarma' trades the threat of sickness for the promise of health's return.

In both 'SIDA: Crece la alarma' and 'Alarma: El virus que viene de California', whatever threat HIV/AIDS may pose to Spanish society is immediately negated by soothing comments from the medical and social structures of the time, which enforce a political narrative of the general (and perpetual) health of the state. The danger to the figural and literal child could be consequently minimized as belonging to a very small and controlled subset of medical anomalies, as well as through a renewed insistence on the boundless vitality and health of childhood. The sexualized nature of the illness, however, like the very real physical threat of AIDS, could not be completely neutralized by any amount of medical or political reassurances. Further, the 'risk' of children's sexuality suggested by their contact with this illness clearly motivates many of the television reports seen below, which scramble to normalize childhood and recuperate its conservative promise of the status quo.

It should be stressed that the figural child's promise is conservative inasmuch as it reifies existing structures of power and inequality while promoting normative sex and procreative heterosexuality. The future that such common configurations of childhood offer, then, enables certain social disparities and discourages sexual alterities that do not actively serve to maintain or promote the essentiality of youth. As I explore in this chapter, illness—and in particular, HIV/AIDS—may be a way to circumvent the static forms of childhood currently in play. The representations of infected children that are examined below offer a way out of the generational circularity of the future; through them, I see the struggling articulation of what it means to live through the traumatic event of an emerging epidemic, or what it means to articulate a structure of feeling sick. This articulation—multivocal and barely formed—also helps to imagine a figural child that can invigorate the stale discourses surrounding AIDS, illness, and even sex.[8] In sum, I find myself returning to possibilities—to the sometimes fragile structures of feeling that emerge from living through the event of history-in-the-making and to the potential of an illness like HIV/AIDS to make us uncomfortable with the existing narratives that keep the kid healthy, the queer sick, and the future the same.

Kathryn Bond Stockton's assertion of the 'inherent queerness' of childhood is thus useful for reclaiming some of the potential that may be lost in current conceptualizations of childhood. For Stockton, the queerness of childhood is made apparent in a number of ways, not the least of which occurs in the form of the child who we retroactively think of as gay.[9] Instead, what queers all children (and not just the proto-gay ones) is our assignation of innocence to them, which makes them both strange and appealing (Stockton 2009, 30). Innocence is thus, for Stockton, 'a form of normative strangeness', a queer state of being that must always be recovered after its loss: 'From the standpoint of adults, innocence is alien, since it is "lost" to the very adults who assign it to children. Adults retrospect it through the gauzy lens of what they attribute to the child' (2009, 30–31). The queerness of childhood, then, lies in its fundamentally undiscoverable nature, which likely neither resembles nor reflects the innocence ascribed to it. The desire to reclaim childhood by reasserting its normative timelines and by

8 Regarding this potential promise: when confronting the realities of disease, it may not be enough to imagine new discourses that risk becoming folded into the powerful mix of innocence and futurity promised by the figure of the child. Embracing the 'bad' promise of AIDS—considering, flinchingly, HIV/AIDS to have any 'promise' at all, in fact—seems tone deaf and discursively dangerous. Part of what has made Edelman's *No Future* so polemical and divisive is his denial of the child's promise that 'tomorrow is only a day away' (2004, 18), and his subsequent call to turn to negativity, queerness, and the death drive, imagining a world without futurity. It is clear, I hope, that this is not the purpose of the current chapter, although my project shares many kinships with Edelman's acceptance of what are commonly considered 'bad objects' and affects, as I discuss in this book's conclusion.

9 Such an appellation is 'retroactive', according to Stockton (2009, 6–7), as it is taken up by others or by oneself and applied after the fact. The queer-identifying adult applies queerness to their childhood, potentially even before the development of fully realized romantic attachments or sexual desire, and thus reconfigures moments of childhood under this queer lens and from the guise of the future looking back on the past.

purifying it from sexuality helps to explain further the father's pressing need to maintain Rafael's innocence (read: ignorance), no matter the psychic damage to himself or his son.

Stockton's ideas are provocative, and guide some of my conclusions about how HIV/AIDS in children came to be represented in the news reports and media of this time in Spain. The cultural and political problem that is animated in these representations, along with the energy expended in presenting the 'true victim' as the child with AIDS, will continually recur throughout this chapter. Is the future established by the figural child so delicate, necessitating such care and maintenance over the child's representation? Or is it, as I assert, that the continual demands that childhood and futurity be tended to and nourished are precisely their strength, that we are enthralled to the very futures we cultivate, and that we are committed to stasis and normativity, perhaps even despite our desires to the contrary? The children portrayed in the following reports are shown to be deserving of our care and affection, and as such they are shielded figures of an epidemic that boasts too many forgotten, discarded, and willfully disregarded individuals. As Stockton writes, 'it is a privilege to need to be protected—and to be sheltered—and thus to have a childhood' (2009, 31). That privilege underscores our upkeep of childhood and our commitment to its sustained purity, both within and because of illness.

Queer bloodlines

The privileges afforded to youth and childhood in the earliest years of Spain's AIDS outbreak are made patently evident in its television news media, which produced a stream of reports on children and AIDS between 1983 and 1987. Most notable among these are episodes of the much-loved health program *Más vale prevenir* (June 16, 1985 and January 9, 1987), the science program *Generación 800* (September 19, 1985), and the variety show *El domingo es nuestro* (March 15, 1987). Together, these programs and reports shape an image of AIDS in its earliest years as intimately tied to youth and childhood, the face of the future in Spain, while demonstrating a desire to safeguard normalcy and health. The end result is an attempt to rewrite the damage wrought by illness for a segment of the population, even as others were left behind in the past.

Written, directed, and hosted by the journalist Ramón Sánchez Ocaña, *Más vale prevenir* debuted in 1979 and ran for eight years on RTVE.[10] In

10 This was not, however, the extent of Sánchez Ocaña's media presence or the end of his work on issues of childhood and youth health. *Más vale prevenir* was followed

that time, it aired special episodes on a wide range of health topics, from tobacco use to hepatitis, hair loss to obesity. As these topics suggest, the show was aimed at a broad audience—one that was both health-conscious and interested in its particular style of educational television—and pledged itself to helping its viewers 'procurar un mañana más sano' [have a healthier tomorrow], as it stated in the earliest iterations of its opening credits. In its quest to address issues of broad public interest as well as emerging health topics and events, it covered the AIDS epidemic twice during its stint on air—once in late 1985, and then in early 1987.[11] In both of these episodes, the program concerned itself with raising general awareness of the illness and dispelling its myths, which is to say that unlike many of the frenzied early reports on HIV and AIDS—those that came before or after, as well as those that originated in Spain or elsewhere—the approach of *Más vale prevenir* to illness was fairly measured and scientifically oriented.

Still, and as I note throughout this book, scientific rigor and measured reporting do not always attract audiences, and even the most purportedly objective of programs is predicated on a desire to deliver its message in an entertaining manner. For *Más vale prevenir,* that message is that its audience be healthy, which is to pointedly say that it not be sick. From this perspective, which seems to be the prevailing viewpoint of health in many modern Western societies, the injunction to 'be healthy' means a host of things, not the least of which is ' be safe'. It also suggests that healthiness is a state to aspire to, a condition of physical normativity that requires upkeep and

by a sister program, *Diccionario de la Salud*, which aired from 1988 to 1989 and was also written, directed, and hosted by Sánchez Ocaña. A special documentary, *Los hijos del frío*, completed Sánchez Ocaña's contract with RTVE on January 7, 1991. Like the shows preceding it, *Los hijos del frío* placed children front and center, reporting on the changing face of reproductive issues due to technological advances in fertilization in vitro and in sperm bank procedures.

11 The fact that these episodes aired early in the outbreak of the epidemic in Spain and that HIV/AIDS was never revisited in either of Sánchez Ocaña's subsequent shows, despite the increasing prominence of the illness in the late 1980s, is unsurprising for any number of reasons: the show's information-based format relied on bringing new guidance on treatment and prevention of common health risks and problems, so perhaps AIDS was seen as being both well-known and untreatable, and therefore no longer so important to audiences. Similarly, the focus on family issues and general health and wellbeing could also preclude revisiting the illness once it had been firmly placed into the realm of niche health issues. In contrast, the timing of the two produced episodes seems to have been designed, as noted in this chapter, to combat misinformation and assuage public fears at key moments in the outbreak—in its initial stages, and on the advent of medical treatment.

continual vigilance. You can become healthy, but only if you follow the right rules; and you can always be healthier, particularly by taking the appropriate measures, as they are outlined in episode after episode. In this manner, then, and by taking the safekeeping of Spanish citizenry as its purpose, *Más vale prevenir* upholds the promise of a healthy (and healthier) tomorrow for present and future citizens.

The directive toward health and futurity is apparent even in the show's opening credits, which changed several times during its run but generally always featured children prominently. In the earliest variation of the credits (1979), images of women and men on sidewalks can be seen, followed by quick jump cuts to bustling streets full of cars intercut with images of legs and people walking. Across the screen, the words 'Radio-televisión Española presenta' [presents] wipe into view. Abruptly, the credits cut to a nurse dressing a little girl in a hospital, and the title text appears on screen. The camera pulls back, revealing a sequence of hospital rooms filled with children in pink being read to, playing with dolls, and lying down in their beds. The jaunty music continues as the credits display scenes of a doctor patting a crying baby and speaking to the camera, children running in circles outside, a child dangerously close to a boiling pot and a close-up of another riding a vacuum cleaner. Childhood is continually at risk in these credits, and children are shown to live on the edge of danger—but this is simultaneously juxtaposed with caring adults who pat them, tend to them, cure them, and pull them away from boiling pots just in time. Better an ounce of prevention, as the idiomatic title suggests, than the wild dangers of unchecked childhood, which are continually fraught with peril in the credits.[12] The opening sequence continues as the camera pans over potentially hazardous household instruments—pointy screwdrivers, small choking hazards, safety pins, and scissors—before cutting back to the open boiling pot and a child rebelliously throwing a paper plane at it. A boy leans over a balcony, high in the sky, and another pushes a chair toward an open window. The children in this opening montage, willfully courting death despite their guardians' best intentions, are unrepentant.[13]

12 The show's title, *Más vale prevenir*, is derived from the Spanish idiom 'Más vale prevenir que curar' [Better to prevent than to cure], which most closely correlates to the English-language idiom 'An ounce of prevention is worth a pound of cure.'

13 As noted earlier, these are only the earliest opening credits of the show, and they were changed a number of times throughout its run. Still, children often retained a place in the opening and closing credits: by 1980 the show was opening with a pair of infants who grow up into children, adolescents, adults, and finally into old age before walking off into the sunset of (presumed) death; by 1983 these credits were replaced with the now-classic sequence of a cartoon man who studiously avoids

As Stockton reminded us earlier, there is a great privilege in needing to be protected and sheltered, which is at its core a description of childhood (2009, 31). Our modern conceptualizations of childhood as fragile and weak, an easily broken state of being that requires constant adult supervision, shapes the way we regard children, and lurks in the guiding ethos of *Más vale prevenir*. Whatever our personal beliefs regarding the care of children—maybe we think they need to get hurt a little to learn and grow, maybe we are protective of their fragility and innocence, or maybe we just don't like them—we tend to regard them as unaware of the world's dangers and thus in need of some sort of sheltering. What Stockton suggests here is thus vital for understanding how boiling water, scissors, balconies, and playgrounds churn with low-level menace in the opening sequence of *Más vale prevenir*, which is that the creation of innocence in childhood necessitates the concomitant creation of adult intercession on its behalf. Applied liberally, that intercession then spills over into those actions, people, or hazards that are then seen as anti-child, inappropriately adult, and dangerous. The threats that stalk childhood, then, can be easily seen to be illness, the unsafe world, and sex and sexuality.

In the early 1980s, AIDS provided that threat in spades. *Más vale prevenir*, primed as it was to spot aberrant threats to the health and wellness of Spain, responded in turn. The first of its episodes on the illness, broadcast on June 16, 1985, was 'dedicado al SIDA, estudiando su historia y dando recomendaciones para evitarlo, también se explica por qué es conveniente respirar por la nariz y qué hacer frente a la tensión de los exámenes' [dedicated to AIDS, studying its history and giving recommendations on avoiding it, also explaining why it is best to breathe through one's nose, and how to combat the stress of exams], according to the episode's timing transcript. This assortment of themes was common to most episodes of *Más vale prevenir*, serving to show just how the program shuffled increasingly deadly epidemics into the mundaneness of life events—like school exam periods or proper breathing techniques. In a similar fashion, the casual juxtaposition of these topics makes clear that the show's audience was not in fact the groups who were perceived to be most at risk, but those that could afford to only briefly turn their attention to AIDS before fretting over how to deal with their children's school-related stress or wondering if they were breathing in the most efficient manner; in other words, and broadly speaking, a sober, heterosexual population not currently facing an encroaching epidemic, or at least one that was being actively shielded from its threat.

pitfalls and hazards on his way to work, with closing credits that depict children frolicking in a meadow, the promise of protected youth.

As a relatively early[14] broadcast in Spain on AIDS, the 1985 episode of *Más vale prevenir* spends the majority of its segment substantiating the threat to certain 'risk groups', a practice discussed in Chapter 1 as one that effectively isolated the threat of the illness from the population at large. Beginning by discussing how difficult it is to talk about AIDS since so little is known about it, Sánchez Ocaña states that the illness 'se puede definir [...] como una alteración grave en el sistema defensivo del individuo ... Esta definición partía de que no se sabía el origen. Hoy, sin embargo, parece claro que el origen está precisamente aquí—' [can be defined ... as a deadly alteration in an individual's defensive system ... This definition came from the fact that its origin was unknown. Today, nevertheless, it seems clear that the origin is precisely here—] (Sánchez Ocaña 1985). Abruptly ending his sentence in suspense, Sánchez Ocaña points toward the camera, a movement that also points to the viewing audience, as if for a second to frame the origins of the virus as localizable within them. Before this might be fully processed by any audience member, however, a pre-taped segment begins. The viewer can heave a sigh of relief, feeling comforted that they are not the cause, that a virus is the villain here, and that this culprit can be seen and understood. Perhaps it seems frivolous to note this moment, a common trick in television and film that relies on the viewer's ability to recognize shots and reverse shots as conforming to the dynamic of a spoken dialogue, but it is precisely this moment that captures the spirit of Sánchez Ocaña's initial treatment of AIDS, which can seemingly only affect a certain populace under special conditions, and which its television viewer will never contract. The seemingly slight gesture, then, turns into a sleight of hand: you briefly had AIDS, and now I've made it disappear. In its place is a virus, the culprit and enemy.

A virus is a nebulous, moving target, however, and its ability to hide out in the body complicates the way it is often perceived; that is to say, as discussed throughout this book, a virus is at once part of one's self and foreign to it, a complex knot of otherness with which we often maintain a hesitant relationship. At the risk of overstating what at this point may be patently evident, the easiest enemies to pin blame on were the classic categories upon which the majority of AIDS history rests: drug users and homosexuals. As the episode continues, it turns to the chief microbiologist of the National

14 As seen in other chapters, though there were reports on HIV/AIDS in Spanish print media as early as late 1981, there were no major televised reports on the illness until the May 14, 1983 episode of *Informe semanal*. As news of the discovery of HIV was still being reported and its possible modes of contagion were still debated, the year 1985 thus represents a relatively early visual representation of the illness on Spanish television, despite its chronological delay otherwise.

Centre for Microbiology in Spain, Asia de la Loma Danilova, whose remarks follow the now-established outbreak narrative for Spain (and much of the Western world):

> [El SIDA] se presentaba en los principios de la enfermedad en grupos de homosexuales que tenían muchas parejas en sus relaciones sexuales, en grupos de drogadictos que se inoculaban intravenosamente y usando normalmente jeringas compartidas—y también se presentaba como grupo de riesgo en los hemofílicos, pero en una proporción muy pequeña. (Sánchez Ocaña 1985)[15]

De la Loma's remarks need little parsing at this point, as they follow the routine discourse of condemnation of sexuality and drug use among the purported risk groups of AIDS, seen throughout this book so often that it becomes a near-mantra for the early years of the epidemic in Spain. Here the remarks are notable, however, as they mark the 'bad adults' in the narrative constructed by *Más vale prevenir*—the ones who stand in the way of the growth of happy, healthy childhood, who represent a threat to national promises of futurity. The deviant adults here—the bearers of bad sexuality, the ones addicted to life-damaging drugs—are the antithesis of those who pull children away from scalding pots and rescue the ones on the balcony. They court death, reject the future, and embrace illness with bad practices.

After spending some time on the segments of the populace who do find themselves in danger, Sánchez Ocaña ends his report on AIDS by discussing the children of infected drug addicts who become HIV-positive and must be hospitalized. For the average spectator, it may feel like an uneasy way to end the report, summing up quickly how the negative actions of the few affect a new group of people—children—who are now forever tainted. But by that same token, it must feel logical, this leap; the camera trick that threatened the viewer with illness turned its kino eye instead to the still images of a virus, and finally to the moving images of those whose bad practices court death and put childhood in danger. In the logic of this move, then, childhood is always the underlying knot to worry over, constantly in danger from the physical world and stalked by the shadowy figure of the sick stranger. Those who value the future, *Más vale prevenir* suggests, must keep childhood safe.

By the show's second episode on AIDS in 1987, the illness had revealed itself to be even more widespread and threatening than imagined just two

15 '[AIDS] emerged in groups of homosexuals who had a lot of sexual partners, in groups of drug addicts who normally injected themselves with shared needles—also another risk group emerged in hemophiliacs, although as a very small percentage.'

years earlier. In contrast to the previous episode, the entire running time of the 1987 airing was spent discussing the spread of AIDS in a roundtable with medical experts on the illness. After Sánchez Ocaña has presented the special guests in attendance, the program cuts to a brief sequence from the 1985 episode. Upon returning to the roundtable, the presenter notes:

> Hoy evidentemente las circunstancias han cambiado. El tema ha cobrado muchísima más actualidad. Ya saben ustedes que hace poco el consejo de Europa destinó una importante cantidad de dinero para la prevención, incluso en EE. UU. están haciendo campañas importantísimas para la prevención e información de todos los ciudadanos. Y se llega a decir que en el año 2000 va a haber alrededor de 100 millones de enfermos del SIDA. El tema es lo suficientemente importante como para abordarlo y por eso hemos invitado a estar con nosotros a una serie de cualificados especialistas. (Sánchez Ocaña 1987)[16]

Perhaps what is most striking here are the 'changed circumstances' that Sánchez Ocaña seeks to highlight in these opening remarks, which are exclusively changes in perception of the virus from the perspective of the purportedly healthy majority. In other words, the virus hasn't actually changed in this time period, nor has its innate inability to infect others—yet a wider public is now aware and afraid of the illness, there is greater discussion of cases that fall outside the narrowly defined risk groups, and some government action has begun to lumber forward, however halting and feeble. These are significant changes, but by no means do they represent any sort of systemic shift in the way that homosexuals, drug users, and hemophiliacs—for starters—were made to bear the representative force of the illness in its early years. In short, the privilege of ignoring the breathtakingly devastating losses from HIV/AIDS for six years is clearly lost to Sánchez Ocaña in this moment.

This moment marks a significant tonal shift from the 1985 episode, which bracketed the concern around HIV/AIDS with the breezy suggestion that not only would the audience not be affected by the illness, but that they might be safekeepers of health and wellness for their children. No such promise is

16 'Today, evidently, circumstances have changed. The topic has become increasingly more current. You all already know that recently the Council of Europe earmarked a significant amount of money for its prevention, and in the United States they are running very important campaigns on prevention and the information of all of its citizens. It's even being said that by the year 2000 there will be around 100 million sick from AIDS. The topic is sufficiently important to take on, and so we have invited a number of qualified specialists to be with us.'

made here, not when concerns for general public health have piqued fears so sharply. Also differing in this episode is Sánchez Ocaña himself, who was so often the calm voice of reason in *Más vale prevenir*, capable of patiently allaying dramatic fears over a broad range of illnesses or actions, and carefully nudging his viewership toward being better informed about their health and wellness. Instead, Sánchez Ocaña seems genuinely uninformed during this episode, peppering with a crude joke or two questions that teeter dangerously on the edge of homophobia, racism, and dangerous misinformation.

Perhaps we shouldn't be surprised at this tone or Sánchez Ocaña's affect, or at least not completely; after all, many of the questions he asks during the roundtable might still be asked today by someone somewhere, a person aggressively stuck in the belief that their health is being encroached upon by an illness that should be reserved for a small cadre of undesirables. If anything, however, it is precisely the well-meaning ignorance of the host that should cause worry, along with his responsibility to relay a series of good health practices. Standing in for the uninformed mass that represents his straight, white, and sober viewing audience, then, seems like the real risky practice here, as he voices prejudices and common misunderstandings with no real medical truths behind them.

Despite the host's casual cluelessness, the ensuing roundtable debate and its team of medical panelists do their best to dispel some of the stigma around the illness. The panel included Dr. Emilio Gómez de la Concha (Chief of the Division of Immunology at the Hospital Clínico de Madrid), Dr. Antonio García Pérez (Professor of Dermatology at the Universidad Complutense de Madrid), Dr. Julio Rodríguez Villanueva (Professor of Microbiology at the Universidad de Salamanca), and Dr. Rafael Nájera (Director of the Instituto de Salud Carlos III). These medical figures—immunologists, virologists, microbiologists, and even a dermatologist—deflect a range of common misconceptions and beliefs about the viral origins and transmission of HIV/AIDS during the show's thirty-minute episode. When the host asks about the most 'normal' transmission method for HIV/AIDS, for example, García Pérez responds by noting that the globally common risk factors of homosexuality and drug use are also present in Spain, but with drug users becoming infected at a much higher rate. Ultimately, he states, it boils down to the fact that 'en España el problema del SIDA actualmente es sobre todo un problema de transmisión por drogas' [in Spain, the problem of AIDS is currently (and) above all else a problem of transmission through drugs] (Sánchez Ocaña 1987). Like many newscasters and public figures before him, and in tune with the general discourse of the time, Sánchez Ocaña is insistent in the overlap of the two groups, stressing that 'muchos drogadictos se prostituyen' [a lot of drug addicts prostitute themselves]. García Pérez shrugs the remark off, concluding: 'En ocasiones, sí, pero no en todos casos. Son dos mundos distintos' [Ocassionally, yes, but not in every case. They're separate worlds] (Sánchez Ocaña 1987).

There is much more to say about this episode and about moments like this when the mention of homosexuality slides into a discussion of prostitution, but that is just one of a number of issues: for example, when Sánchez Ocaña jokingly ruminates on the urban myths that fueled some of the earliest conspiracies around AIDS—from its creation in a lab to its potential extra-terrestrial origins—or when he asks why AIDS has emerged at this precise moment, in its plague-like form, when there are so many carriers in Africa. The first question gives some small credence to conspiracy theory over medical knowledge, while the second presupposes that the status of 'plague' is only conferred when a European populace is affected; as such both questions are woefully ignorant from a person who was such an important medical figure at the time (for, regardless of medical training, this is precisely what Sánchez Ocaña was). These questions are even more striking given Sánchez Ocaña's own book on the epidemic, *Ante el SIDA: ¿Qué puedo hacer?*, which was published the very same year.

One of the most interesting of these moments comes at the end of this episode, when Sánchez Ocaña begins to make his closing statements. Speaking of the rise of AIDS-related cases among children, he closes: 'Hay sesenta y dos. La mayoría pertenece a hijos de enfermos del SIDA. Veintinueve son hijos de madres drogadictas, dieciséis eran hemofílicos y doce habían recibido transfusiones de sangre' [There are sixty-two. The majority of these belong to children of people with AIDS. Twenty-nine are children of drug addicts, sixteen were hemophiliacs and twelve had received blood transfusions] (Sánchez Ocaña 1987).[17] As in his 1985 episode, Sánchez Ocaña ends this segment abruptly by turning to childhood and children with HIV/AIDS. It is difficult to know the precise reasoning behind this closing statement, which merely informs the viewing audience but provides no context or discussion. Unlike the earlier episode, the focus is no longer merely on the children of drug users but on the method of transmission and the numbers of children who have been affected by the virus. What is clear is that the end result is another uneasy sendoff, another closing statement that brackets the discussion of risk groups and bad practices in order to focus on figures of innocence and futurity.

17 Like nearly every attempt to provide accurate case counts during this period, the numbers of children with AIDS that Sánchez Ocaña lists here are debatable. The potential for miscounting is understandable, for a multitude of reasons: the soft borders between childhood and adolescence being one possibility, as is the unknown number of unreported cases where patients died without being properly diagnosed.

This moment is important because it refuses to let the viewer forget whose lives really matter, and what exactly the damaging effects of the illness are—not, in other words, the quibbling over how many prostitute drug addicts are out terrorizing the streets, nor which part of Africa is most responsible for the plague on the public's doorstep. The latter are clearly important issues for Sánchez Ocaña (particularly in his mission to educate a broad segment of the population on issues of health and wellness), but his concern lies squarely with the near future. By closing in this manner, he seems to insist that we must never let go of the imperative to safeguard that future, always reaching for a better and healthier tomorrow through the figure of the child.

In the blood

At the root of the fear for the infected child is the sense that his blood, so important to the sustained dream of the nation, has been irrevocably tampered with. It might have been easier to dismiss HIV/AIDS when it was believed to be a product of aberrant sex or uncontrolled drug use, but its spread into the Spanish blood supply fanned the fear that this mysterious illness could be lurking anywhere—in the veins of your neighbor, a friend, or the kid in the playground. Following the initial portrayal of AIDS as a hemophiliac child's disease in Spanish media and the subsequent (and immediate) quelling of panic by news outlets and governmental sources alike, the reports that eventually turned to portraying the child as exemplary AIDS victim from 1985 onwards corroborated fears that the illness had now infected the futurity of the nation. As seen in *Más vale prevenir* and the news articles discussed above, the number of newly infected children meant that the national future could no longer exist as promised, tainted as it now was, and suggested that personal futures might likewise be destabilized. This realization was, of course, not entirely novel to the Spanish public, who had not only lived through the illnesses resulting from the years of hunger during the Franco dictatorship but had even more recently seen a rise in hepatitis cases and the appearance of Toxic Oil Syndrome in the years immediately preceding the advent of HIV/AIDS. The particular impact of this illness, however, was tied to its unknowability and its mystery, themselves products of long incubation periods and rapid physical decline. The result of HIV's introduction into the bloodstream of Spain seemed to be to contaminate the blood of the nation—in ways that were at once literal and deeply metaphorical.

Like the figural importance given to the heart and the mind as seats of intelligence and emotion, discussions of the blood in our bodies have often conjured up a host of symbols corresponding to life and death, health and illness, and the sustained promise of the national body. Feldman and Bayer, for example, write how the colors, flow, scientific properties, and social significance of blood have long contributed to the symbolic power that it holds over a collective cultural imagination (1999, 2). They add that it 'has been viewed as the apogee of purity and the nadir of filth; cited as both the basis for unity and justification for war; analyzed as a gift that brings life and a source of death; and sold as a commodity that has been called priceless' (1999, 2). Dorothy Nelkin, examining the development of cultural perspectives on blood, describes it as both an 'objective, biological substance' and 'a cultural entity with complex social meanings that vary in different cultures and change over time' (1999, 274–75). In a similar vein, and writing on the potential for violence inherent in a cultural imaginary of blood, Robert Esposito theorizes that blood is 'salvific for the all *inasmuch as* it is destructive to a part. It has the capacity to cleanse *just as* it is meant to soil. It generates life *because* it causes death' (2011, 39). In the passages above, Esposito, Nelkin, and Feldman and Bayer highlight the cultural weight attributed to issues of blood and its metaphors, and in so doing they challenge the simple perception of blood as mere physical substance and medical object.

As discussed in the introduction, Lina Meruane's *Viral Voyages* turns to local meanings of blood, thinking through blood metaphors of Latin America in order to accentuate the fluidity of AIDS discourse and transmission and describing how the circumstances of the illness's origins are part of a larger global condition that prizes liquidity and movement. Citing Steven Epstein, she uses the language of mobile capital and globalization to discuss the 'infectious language of leakage and containment' (qtd in Meruane 2014, 17–18) in which AIDS is often couched, which clearly leans on the symbolic sense of blood (and other concurrent bodily processes) to convey a sense of the national. Of the infectious spread of AIDS, she notes how

> the virus, according to medicine's authoritative discourse, does not just penetrate [the] system but also multiplies rapidly within its cells until they explode, spreading out again through the body, which is more and more defenseless, and transmitting itself to others. This destructive operation is carried out through bodily *fluids*—blood, semen, saliva, tears—fluids that are very much of a piece with the new semantics of the economic system. (Meruane 2014, 17–18)

It becomes evident just how the system of global metaphors of blood come to be utilized in a variety of ways. For Meruane, of course, this is not simply about blood but water travel, other bodily fluids, the economic 'trickle-down' policies of the 1980s, and even the understanding of globalization as a fluid concept.

Far from expressing confusion over what blood can mean, these ideas navigate global and local environments, demonstrating just how many meanings blood can have, along with how culturally fluid these meanings are. The multivalence behind the way we imagine and react to blood has deep ramifications for ostensibly neutral or factual accounts of blood. That is, how can we imagine that blood is a substance with which only medical institutions have made meaning? Nelkin lists many such meanings and metaphors, few of which belong exclusively to the terrain of the medical, instead shaping our cultural perceptions of nations, communities, race, and gender:

> Blood is seen as a source of life and energy, but it is also a symbol of violence and danger. It is a metaphor for social solidarity and the connection between the individual and society, but it has also represented the biological distinctions between people and is linked to the politics of race and social class. Blood is a social fluid that calls for altruistic relationships, but blood plasma is an economic product that can be competitively bought and sold. Purity of blood is a clinical concept associated with physical health, but it is also a racist construct used to define ethnicity and justify exclusivity and discrimination. (1999, 275)

This description of blood shows the difficulty of fixing any one particular meaning to the substance, although it was in large part due to the types of values that have been attached to blood that the numbers of infected hemophiliacs became so high in Spain. The meanings and metaphors ascribed to it weigh heavily in discussions of quarantine, guilt, shame, innocence, risky actions, and healthy and sick bodies. As such, the introduction of a foreign agent—the germ, virus, or illness—into the national pipeline of a bloodstream taints what is an ostensibly pure domestic fount of civic energy and identity.

In the discussions of HIV/AIDS that center around hemophiliacs (and indeed, as we will see it repeated with each so-called AIDS risk group), infected blood is a mark, one that denotes the carrier as outside the defensible borders of the nation. Infected blood means a loss of immunity ascribed to those within our national body politic, a loss of place within the confines of the healthy national community, and a loss of social status. As Nelkin notes,

> until the seventeenth century work of William Harvey, people commonly attributed disease to bad blood. But, also, it was widely believed that the biological properties of blood varied with the social position of the person. Nobles, for example, enjoyed superior social status because of the purity of their blood and the integrity of their bloodline. (1999, 284)

The concept of social attribution formulated through 'good' or 'bad' blood is wholly apparent within the literature of and around the HIV/AIDS epidemic, as it was also apparent in the eugenics movements of the nineteenth and twentieth centuries in Spain and elsewhere, which defined healthy nationalism as an encounter with healthy or sick citizens' bodies. Alfredo Sosa-Velasco underscores the importance of eugenics in Spain in the early twentieth century by noting how 'la eugenesia definió las distinciones biológicas y culturales de género, y la raza y el género se construyeron a partir de imágenes y prácticas sociales que encajaran dentro de la nación' [eugenics defined biological and cultural distinctions of gender, and race and gender were built up from images and social practices that fit within the concept of the nation] (2010, 65). The popularity of eugenics crafted a system where difference is boiled down to blood. The concurrent eugenic belief in the biological roots of mental, cultural, and social variation between persons likewise allows for the reduction of difference to hereditary traits, passed down generationally.

Such generational reproduction, in turn, further underscores the heterosexual nature of our blood metaphors and their ties to cultural products. As Sosa-Velasco writes, the marriage of race and eugenics creates and promotes

> el deseo de 'imaginar' la nación en términos biológicos, de 'purificar' la reproducción de las poblaciones para que encajen en las normas de la herencia, de regular el flujo de los habitantes dentro de las fronteras nacionales, y de definir bajo términos nuevos quiénes pertenecen a la nación y quiénes no. (2010, 65)[18]

18 '[T]he desire to "imagine" the nation in biological terms, to "purify" the reproductive habits of populations so that these fit hereditary norms, to regulate the flow of those who live within national borders, and to define under new terms who belongs to the nation and who does not.' There is much more to say about eugenics than can be expressed here, chiefly the very real possibility that some lingering aspects of a belief in a pure, nationalized bloodline might still remain in Spanish popular thought, exacerbated by German and Francoist discourse of the mid-twentieth century and the decades of dictatorship which highlighted and

Spain's history with eugenics has undoubtedly shaped some of the cultural power of blood in the conceptualization of HIV/AIDS. What's more, and as was the case under eugenics and the conceptualizations of community and immunity it created, HIV and hemophilia have been routinely seen as more than the sum of their parts; that is, infection or illness with either becomes representative of a lack of power, national and individual weakness, congenital and racial defectiveness, and general deviance.[19]

Hemophiliacs in Spain already understood all too well the significance of blood as both a lifegiving and a destructive force. As one of the first groups in Spain to be affected by the spread of HIV, however, they quickly found themselves forced to undergo a new process by which their illness was recast as cultural defect, capable of inducing moral panic and judgment. Perhaps precisely for that reason, the conclusion of 'Alarma: El virus que viene de California' turns to the effects of the illness within the hemophiliac community. As theorized both here and in Chapter 1, this turn is a way to contain AIDS while providing a palliative response to the threat to the larger body politic. The report's concluding segment provides a brief statement by Enrique de Galinsoga, the Secretary General of the Asociación Española de Hemofílicos [Spanish Hemophiliac Association]. At the start of the AIDS outbreak, as Galinsoga remarks, about 90% of Spain's plasma (used in the treatment of hemophilia) was imported from the United States, with the remaining 10% acquired from altruistic donations within Spain. Although the association was in the midst of what would turn out to be a very complex and lengthy set of negotiations with the Spanish government to create their own plasma donation centers (and therefore no longer receive potentially infected plasma from American-based companies), Galinsoga also firmly states that hemophiliacs have nothing to worry about. His statements give credence to a common belief of the time, which is that unlike the seemingly chaotic nature of homosexuality (either in its promiscuity or unruliness),

racialized xenophobia. It is beyond the scope of this book to probe this line of thought too deeply, so instead I signal others who have discussed eugenics and issues of national health in Spain, notably *The Spanish Flu: Narrative and Identity in Spain, 1918* (Davis 2013) and *Deaf History and Culture in Spain: A Reader of Primary Documents* (Fraser 2009).

19 Tuberculosis is, perhaps, the most obvious example of a blood disease with a long history of symbolic representations in literature—most often seen as a romantic's disease from the seventeenth century onward, or as reflecting a body too full of passions in nineteenth-century literature. For more information, Sontag (1990) provides an incisive juxtaposition and overview of the differing representations of cancer and tuberculosis; Byrne (2011) and Lawlor (2006) discuss the role of tuberculosis and gender in English literature; and Woodard, Joyce, and McBride (2014) critique its frequently referenced connections to race.

hemophilia can be understood, controlled medically, and quarantined from the general public. That is, until it threatens to break out of this confining narrative, as we will see shortly.

The outbreak of HIV/AIDS among hemophiliacs (both in Spain and worldwide) has a different history to its spread among other populations, as one might imagine. In the introduction and in Chapter 1, I offered a look at the development of HIV/AIDS in Spain, but it is worth examining the specifics of its spread among hemophiliacs in these critical years, as this serves as a backdrop to the reports and films that followed. A year after the earliest known cases of HIV/AIDS were documented, the *Mortality and Morbidity Weekly Report* (*MMWR*) published findings that described some of the first known cases of *Pneumocystis carinii* (a rare type of pneumonia with links to the weakened immune systems of AIDS patients) in hemophiliacs with no other underlying diseases.[20] The report, published in 1982 as '*Pneumocystis carinii* Pneumonia among Persons with Hemophilia A', is significant as it provides early evidence for the presence of HIV in the blood and beyond the established risk groups associated with AIDS. After noting that all three patients were heterosexual males with no history of intravenous drug use, the article summarizes their characteristics, the chronologies of their infections, and (for two of the three) their deaths. An editorial note at the end of the report clarifies its most important findings:

> The clinical and immunologic features these three patients share are strikingly similar to those recently observed among certain individuals from the following groups: homosexual males, heterosexuals who abuse IV drugs, and Haitians who recently entered the United States. Although the cause of the severe immune dysfunction is unknown, the occurrence among the three hemophiliac cases suggests the possible transmission of an agent through blood products. (Centers for Disease Control and Prevention 1982b, n.p.)

Pointing to the patients' hemophilia, the report further surmises a potential common culprit to all three patients—their treatment for Factor VIII deficiencies. Factor VIII is a blood-clotting protein whose deficiency in hemophiliacs forms the basis of their illness; its lack is treated through intravenous injections which—at the time—were produced in one of two

20 According to a passing mention in another *MMWR* article, 'Update: Acquired Immunodeficiency Syndrome (AIDS) in Persons with Hemophilia', an earlier case of HIV/AIDS and hemophilia was reported in 1981 (Centers for Disease Control and Prevention 1984, n.p.), although it provides no further information or sources for this statement.

ways: through cryoprecipitate (the residue of freshly frozen plasma) or as a concentrate manufactured from plasma pools that had been 'collected from as many as a thousand or more donors' (Centers for Disease Control and Prevention 1982b, n.p.).

The hemophiliac's reliance on exogenous plasma means that countries must either produce their own blood supplies or import them in order to supply treatment, and the differing blood donation systems across countries reveal cultural and medical practices that are often oppositional. It is interesting to see, for example, how a reliance on blood product (different from the so-called 'whole' blood of transfusions, for example) puts into question where national community lines begin and end. Feldman and Bayer note this problem, drawing attention to the fact that

> as blood plasma is increasingly subject to transformation by pharmaceutical firms, it is difficult to sustain the symbolic attachments evoked by whole blood. So too is it difficult to preserve the centrality of the whole blood donor when plasma donation requires a kind of "professional" commitment in both time and effort that is hardly compatible with ... amateur voluntarism. (1999, 8)

Perhaps the blurred boundaries between donor and recipient, or between whole blood and its plasma product, are responsible for the sharp withdrawal into hypernationalism on a sanguineous level, producing a demand for a system of blood autarky, to loosely borrow from Feldman and Bayer (1999, 9). Indeed, as they note, even 'in an era of globalization, in which national borders increasingly give way to regional and international economic forces, both international and national health authorities continue to regard self-sufficiency as the fundamental principle of blood policy' (1999, 9).

The outcomes of so-called blood autarky (or its lack) are vast, and produce ripples of cultural meaning for representations and treatment of blood in visual culture. This is to underscore yet again that blood has already been subject to heavy metaphorization in popular and medical culture; drawing sharp lines around national bloodlines versus foreign blood, along with who belongs to the healthy nation and who will exist outside of it, had profound meaning at the outset of the HIV/AIDS epidemic and still exerts an effect today. In the early years of the epidemic, the debate surrounding blood autarky raged fiercely among hemophiliacs, who saw themselves as victims of a system that prized foreign products over national health. Some of the arguments put forward in the debate over national blood banks, then, capitalized on the belief in blood autarky, a movement that had the potential to shift cultural beliefs or values and affect real outcomes in shaping policies and laws. Yet not all these possibilities had good outcomes, as Feldman and Bayer argue:

> International dependence rather than national self-sufficiency might diminish the sense of belonging to a community in which blood freely circulates as a common currency; it might diminish the willingness to donate; it could result in shortages not remediable through local action; the effectiveness of local regulatory control could be reduced; and injuries or accidents caused by 'foreign' blood could lead to accusation and recrimination infused with racism and xenophobia. (1999, 9)

In pointing to the ways that external blood sources can shift local donation practices, blood bank reserves, and legal processes, Feldman and Bayer demonstrate the cultural import and weight given to blood and blood products. This significance, in turn, has deep through lines to the act of blood donation, which is often seen as a lifegiving sort of altruism in the best of circumstances. Seeking remuneration for blood donation, however, is looked upon far less kindly.

The perception of altruistic donation as opposed to paid is clearly seen in an article by Kate Dunn in the *Canadian Medical Association Journal*, in which she unequivocally states that 'the problem with Factor VIII made from American blood is that the American supply often comes from those most likely to be infected with HIV or other viruses: prostitutes, intravenous drug users and other people in need of quick cash who get it by selling blood' (1993, 612). Dunn is able to make these comments by contrasting Canadian blood donors (who primarily donate altruistically or voluntarily) with American donors, who voluntarily donate less and are more often remunerated for their donations. By dismissing paid donors as those in 'need of quick cash', Dunn sets up a classed dichotomy that distinguishes monetary need from altruistic donation, sharply dividing poverty, sexual deviance, and drug use from altruistic good—and thus separating out those citizens who enact a desire to 'do good' in which money is not, as she reasons, so desperately 'needed'. Strongly splitting these camps of citizens along national lines (good, innocent Canadians versus drug-addled, oversexed Americans) poses a hierarchy of one donation system over another. This in turn allows Dunn to underscore the fact that infected blood product came from donors in the United States and subsequently infected Canadian patients.

Dunn goes on to cite the Canadian Hemophiliac Society, which asserted that 'it has been known for many years that the blood collected from voluntary donors in Canada contains fewer harmful viruses than blood collected from paid donors in the US' (1993, 612). The belief in the inherent goodness of blood donated altruistically—and the correlated 'bad blood' donated for financial gain or out of need—creates a facile dichotomy that has blinded many to the inherent transmissibility of HIV in *all* blood and forms ethical and moral assumptions that are now firmly attached to blood donation. In Spain, where commercial (remunerated) blood donation has long been banned, altruistic donation is only ever painted in terms of solidarity and as evidence of the donor's good character. For example, in a 1982 issue of *Nueva Imagen*, a small graphic relies on solidarity and altruism as the only true path to health. Discussing the treatment procedure for the typical hemophiliac, the article writes that 'el afectado de hemofilia necesita recibir factor VIII o IX para su tratamiento. Ahí es donde debemos colaborar todos nosotros, mediante la donación de nuestra sangre y nuestro plasma' [the person affected by hemophilia needs to receive Factor VIII or IX for his treatment. This is where we have to work together, by way of the donation of our blood and our plasma] (Villace 1982, 7). Framing donation as collaboration, as a solidarity-building act of communitarian labor, is a means by which the hemophiliac community in Spain could construct more unified—or more importantly, accordingly to this logic, healthier—communities.

The image directly below Villace's statement hews to this impulse closely: five large teardrop-shaped images (which are likely meant to be read as blood drops) are arranged in a circle, each with a single word written on them. One-way arrows direct the reading of this organizational outline, so that 'Community' leads to '[Blood] Donation', which leads to 'Transfusions', which leads to 'Industrialization', and finally to 'Services', which connects back up to 'Community' and begins the cycle again. Underneath the image is a small caption: '"Vivir con la Hemofilia". Ayudarnos todos y ayudar a la comunidad' ['Living with Hemophilia': Helping one another and helping the community] (Villace 1982, 7). Connecting the slightly nebulous category of 'services' to community implies that what emerges from industrialization (of blood or otherwise) will benefit not just the sick but the healthy; the community writ large then pays it forward, as it were, which presumably means that a group of healthy citizens enacts its goodness onto the sick by way of blood donation.

To be clear, we have not outgrown these notions of proper communities, altruism, and good blood. On the January 2017 webpage of the Servicio Madrileño de Salud, such goodness is clearly laid out and made explicit under a section titled '¿Por qué debemos donar?' [Why should we donate?] The association cites '10 razones para donar sangre' [10 reasons to donate blood], half of which recur to notions of altruism and generosity that ostensibly make the reader feel better about himself: 'Por solidaridad, altruismo, generosidad ... Porque mañana tú o tus hijos podéis necesitar una donación ... Porque no hay mejor donativo ... Porque con una donación puedes salvar tres vidas ... Porque hay alguien que lo está esperando' [For solidarity, altruism, generosity ... Because tomorrow you or your children may need a donation ... Because there is no better gift ... Because one donation can save three lives ... Because someone is waiting for it] (Servicio Madrileño de Salud n.d.). The belief in 'good blood' (and the correlative ethics of giving blood that emerge from it) had an immediate impact on HIV/AIDS policy, giving rise to some incredible statements by medical professionals in the early years of the epidemic.

In 'Alarma: El virus que viene de California', to take an example, one of the physicians surmises that the diagnosis of AIDS within the hemophiliac community of Spain means that the disease is immediately controllable, while a second, Dr. Castro Artigas, concludes that the city's altruistic donations of blood will nullify the risk of further infection through transfusions. Castro Artigas further surmises that, since all blood and plasma is donated altruistically, 'no existe el menor riesgo' [there is no risk whatsoever] of a further or sustained outbreak among hemophiliacs ('Alarma: El virus que viene de California' 1983).[21] Underscoring these statements is a clear belief in the purity of altruistic blood donations, combating the tainted blood of commercial US plasma and blood product that Spanish hemophiliacs were receiving. In reality, nothing was verifiably safe, and all blood was 'risky', as both of the then-available treatments using Factor VIII turned out to facilitate the transmission of HIV: the multiple, often anonymous and therefore untraceable American donors of blood plasma who donated before effective HIV-screening measures had been established or even invented, and the lack of enhanced purification procedures for the plasma itself.

21 '[Tenemos] la satisfacción de aclarar que, gracias a la colaboración de los 98,000 donantes de sangre como existen en nuestra ciudad, toda cuanta sangre, plasma, plaquetas, glóbulos, etc., se inyecta o se transfunden a los enfermos que los necesitan, son todos de procedencia altruista, entonces, a través de esta procedencia altruista, no existe el menor riesgo. No existe la más mínima preocupación en cuanto a este síndrome de inmunodeficiencia que venimos estudiando' ['We are happy to clarify that thanks to the collaboration of the 98,000 blood donors that exist in our city, any and all blood, plasma, platelets, blood cells, etc. that are injected or transfused to any sick person in need come entirely out of altruism; because of their altruistic origins, there is no risk whatsoever. We do not have the slightest worry with regards to this immunodeficiency syndrome that we've been studying.'] ('Alarma: El virus que viene de California' 1983).

It should be apparent that efforts to address the AIDS crisis in Spain were deeply complicated—when not outright hindered—by attitudes toward blood and blood autarky. These attitudes were further complicated by longstanding beliefs about blood's relationship to purity and national health. On a micro-level, this affected the treatment of individual hemophiliac patients by doctors who heartily supported a hierarchy of blood altruism versus commercialization; on a macro-level, these beliefs altered the very governmental institutions set up to support and protect Spanish citizens. In 1985, Ernest Lluch, the Spanish Minister of Health, appeared on a special 'AIDS episode' of *Generación 800*, a news program that examined current issues in technology and science. In this episode, Lluch spoke about risk groups for AIDS and their effect on adequate treatment of the crisis, while also detailing the status of the illness in Spain and its effect on national blood donation and blood banks. As host Santiago Vázquez describes the calamitous situation facing Spaniards, Lluch responds measuredly:

> Esta situación preocupa, pero lo primero que tendríamos que decir es a quien no debe preocupar. Porque si uno no es drogadicto, si uno no es homosexual o uno no *homofílico* [*sic*], no le debe preocupar. Por lo tanto, la inmensa parte de la población debe estar sosegada puesto que no es población de riesgo. ('EL SIDA' 1985)[22]

Taking a page from the origin story tactics playbook for Spain, Lluch immediately foists the illness onto the prescribed list of bad subjects, the groups who remain the symbolic bearers of AIDS to this day.

It is tempting to push the slip of the tongue aside, ignoring Lluch's conjuring of a *homophiliac* as a simple malapropism born out of the similarity of the *hemo-/homo-* prefixes, or the close proximity of the words in his speech. Doing so, however, obfuscates Lluch's conflation of the figures of the homosexual and the hemophiliac, their fusion into a single group of risky actors responsible for their infections. He was not alone at the time, it should be noted: writing of the proliferations of the word 'homophiliac', Nelkin asserts that it is

> a frequent malapropism that has even been heard in the context of our international meetings involving sophisticated physicians, academics, and administrators involved [in] AIDS policy. It is an amusing slip

22 'This situation is worrisome, but the first thing we have to say is who should not be worried. Because if one is not a drug addict, if one isn't a homosexual or a *homophiliac* [*sic*], it shouldn't worry him. Therefore, the vast majority of the population should feel calmed given that it is not a population at risk.'

> except in the context of the stigmatization of children who test positive for the HIV virus. For they are, inevitably, morally contaminated by their 'bad blood'. (1999, 287)

Unlike Nelkin, I remain less convinced of the inherent humor or amusing nature of the linguistic slip, and instead see it as an example of the symbolic bleed between one risk group and the next. When Lluch states that only these three groups need be concerned, or that the 'vast majority of the population' should be able to rest easy, he effectively pools together a group of sick citizens. The creation of these categories, as I have emphasized repeatedly, has disastrous political, social, and cultural consequences.

What's more, Nelkin's mention of the HIV-positive child as the exceptional AIDS patient returns us to the protected status of innocence and futurity, a state of exception in which children are made guardians of the national (read: pure) bloodline. Along those lines, and while describing the risk that AIDS may or may not pose to the public at large,[23] Lluch continues his interview by stressing the lack of blood autarky in Spain as a decidedly social and ethical issue:

> Nosotros tenemos un España un déficit. De los defectos que tenemos un España, yo diría que uno de los que tenemos es que no damos sangre. Y no dar sangre es un vicio, porque dar algo a los otros gratuitamente es una virtud, y en España damos tres veces menos sangre que el medio europeo. Por lo tanto, primero recomendar a todo el mundo que practiquemos la virtud de dar sangre. ('EL SIDA' 1985)[24]

23 In fact, in Lluch's estimation, the issue that AIDS might pose to Spain is distinctly not grave. Brushing off the lack of political or institutional action by his ministry, he tells Vázquez: 'Decir cosas como lo que yo antes he dicho ... "Bueno, la mayor parte de la población no tiene ningún riesgo" o bien decir algo que es incierto en términos absolutos pero que contiene algo de verdad. El ultimo fin de semana, murieron más españoles en la carretera que españoles han muerto del SIDA desde el año 81' [Saying things like I've just said: 'Well, the better part of the population is not at any risk' or saying something uncertain in absolute terms that nevertheless contains something true. Last weekend, more Spaniards died on the highways than those who have died of AIDS since 81] ('EL SIDA' 1985). Putting aside which number is actually greater, part of the reason Lluch was able to make such an unequivocal claim is, of course, through a very contorted employment of AIDS patients and mortalities that only counts officially diagnosed cases within a very specific timeframe.

24 'In Spain, we have a deficit. Of the defects we have in Spain, I would say one is that we don't give blood. And not giving blood is a vice, because giving something freely to others is a virtue, and in Spain we give three times less blood than the

Citing the national blood bank deficit as a cultural and social 'defect' allows Lluch to couch Spanish blood in moralizing terms; in doing so, donation is set up as a moral decision that is consciously made, and lack of surplus blood product is proof positive of a national 'vice' that is diametrically opposed to the 'virtue' of altruism. He continues by explaining the nationalized system of purchasing blood product from the United States by framing this ethical impasse as brought about by citizens' lack of interest: 'Entonces al no darla, y al no tener además suficiente capacidad industrial, lo que sucede es que importamos plasma sanguíneo de los EEUU, los cuales obtienen de la sangre o bien de países tropicales o bien de colectivos americanos que pasan dificultades sanitarias o de hambre' [So by not giving it, and by not having sufficient industrial capacity either, what happens is that we import blood plasma from the USA, who obtain it from the blood of either tropical countries or from American groups with health issues or hunger] ('EL SIDA' 1985). The United States is a country of great contrasting situations, he explains, so sometimes this blood comes from 'malas circunstancias' [bad circumstances] ('EL SIDA' 1985). He finishes by only obliquely referencing what truly was a blood crisis in Spain, framing it yet again as the product of national vice, rather than poor institutional planning: 'Por lo tanto, esto que podía haber pasado hace tiempo yo creo que en estos momentos no sucede y esperemos que no suceda en el futuro, si cumplimos lo que hemos dictado, si todos trabajamos para que las cosas no solamente se digan sino que se cumplan' [Therefore, what may have happened a little while back no longer happens and we hope won't happen again in the future, if we abide by what we've said, if we all work together so that we don't only say things—we do them] ('EL SIDA' 1985). If an actual crisis could be written off as 'the thing that might have happened a while back' and subsequently reformulated as a national duty with a sharp recrimination to the public (tantamount to wagging a ministerial finger at them), what hope could there be for resolution of the crisis?

Nevertheless, the blood crisis for hemophiliacs did eventually wane, albeit after many, many preventable deaths.[25] As in the 1982 *MMWR* report on the

European average. So I first recommend that we all practice the virtue of giving blood.'

25 Throughout this chapter I have underscored just how these numbers vary wildly, and as such it is difficult to know how many hemophiliacs were infected with HIV in the earliest years of the epidemic in Spain. The most conservative number reported appears in a 1993 article in *El País*, given by the Federación Española de Hemofilia. The number is still, in a word, outrageous. According to the *El País* article, out of 2,730 hemophiliacs receiving plasma treatment, a total of 1,174 tested positive. This is nearly half of all known hemophiliacs in Spain. 416 of those who had been

three HIV-positive hemophiliacs, physicians had warned of the potential for viral transmission through blood products, but it was not until 1983 that procedures were developed to purify blood through pasteurization and chemical means. Like much of the history of HIV/AIDS, however, the global distribution of this treatment was uneven and economically biased. As a result, there were at least four known major corporations that continued to distribute the non-heated (that is, potentially infected) product abroad long after its purified version was made available to patients in the United States (Bogdanich and Koli 2003, n.p.).[26] Although Spain received purified plasma in a fairly timely fashion (and especially compared to other regions like Hong Kong, which received non-treated plasma for several years after 1983), the obligation to analyze plasma was not in place until 1985 with the development of the first HIV antibody test, ELISA (Enzyme Linked Immunosorbent Assay). Such testing was therefore not legally imposed in Spain until October 1985 (Gelabert Blanes 1987, 16). The gaps that set apart the procedural development of treatment for blood (1983), the shipment of purified blood (1983–1985), and the obligation to analyze and treat blood (1985) are wide and created clear inequalities and blood hierarchies. Whose blood mattered, and who truly belonged to the healthy body of the nation? Whose blood was defective, a monstrous threat to society and futurity? These questions animated procedures and laws for years afterward, leaving a trail of bodies behind them as they were debated and discussed in the corridors of hospitals and government buildings.

Treatments

In the first section of this chapter, I pointed to the construction of metaphors around childhood and futurity, how the figure of the child belongs to the promise of a healthy future; through an analysis of some of the earliest news reports and programs around the AIDS epidemic, I also critiqued those instances where childhood was shown as threatened, under attack, and forced out of the national imaginary by way of illness. The fact that such a transformative move—from the expanse of futurity to the foreclosures of mortality—was done through the specter of tainted blood allowed authorities

infected had already succumbed to opportunistic infections, which placed the death rate at about 36% (Criado 1993).

26 These companies were Cutter Biological (a division of Bayer), Armour Pharmaceutical, Baxter International and Alpha Therapeutic. Bogdanich and Koli (2003) and Feldman and Bayer (1999) offer accounts of the purposefully negligent practices behind non-purified Factor VIII global distribution (most often in developing countries).

to exert pressure on existing metaphors of goodness and altruism, virtue and vice, and nationalism and foreign influence. Reigniting the embers of Spanish eugenics, medical and political authorities closed ranks around the purported virtues of national blood, pure and true; toxicity was tied to foreignness, a mysterious viral infection, or an untreated injection of tainted plasma. Childhood was infected by monstrosity.

Of course, such a vision of childhood and futurity supposes that it isn't already tainted by monstrosity, or that we already view children as angelic figures of hope. How do we understand childhood when it has been tainted, queered by something that irrevocably marks the child in some strange way? In some of my earlier work, I drew upon a debate between Judith Butler and Paul Rabinow, in which the two discuss aberrant figures of kinship, statelessness, and liminal personhood. To perhaps oversimplify, what Butler and Rabinow are debating are issues of recognition—who gets recognized by institutional authority and who is refused that privilege, on what terms, and where these acts of recognition or misrecognition occur. As Butler remarks,

> I think there is a zone ... of, say, stateless persons who are and are not persons. And are and are not living, and are and are not recognizable as such. And then the question is how do you go about describing that kind of liminality? And what language is available for that? And what language is available to them? (Butler and Rabinow 2001, 40)

It is apparent to me that these early years of AIDS in Spain set up a hierarchical system of recognition of the sick other—the citizen who is excluded or cared for, the body that is made invisible or rendered as supreme example of altruistic need. Going back to these bodies, lives, and figures and in some small way reclaiming their image from the wreckage of bad institutional policy is one of the most basic endeavors of this book. What Rabinow and Butler are doing here, likewise, reframes this struggle for visibility, thinking through the repercussions of things like the loss of language and voice in these very real struggles of life and death. The AIDS crisis was disastrous for hemophiliacs and, as would be the case for the other risk groups under which they were clustered, so much of the disaster hinged upon issues of their representation in popular media. Following the lead of Butler and Rabinow, however, I want to consider the potential and impact of self-representation as an articulation of feeling sick in a time when so much was unknown. It is a move that can serve at once to flatten difference into normalcy or strategically insert agency into dominant paradigms and institutional strictures. In the case of hemophiliacs, for example, we see a strategy of the former, in which childhood was constantly evoked as a way to destigmatize illness and promote health. Whether this was effective is another matter.

These strategies of representation began early, a few years before the catastrophic introduction of HIV/AIDS into the bloodstream of the Spanish population. In the first issue of the journal *Nueva Imagen*, the president of the Spanish Association of Hemophilia underscored the mission of youth and childhood education as the primary goals behind his association's work. Describing the push for legislation that would positively affect children and adolescents with hemophilia, President José Alonso Gómez wrote: '[propugnamos] que ningún niño en edad escolar quede sin escolarizar, tratando de proporcionarles una orientación escolar y profesional' [we propose that no schoolchildren go without education, in an effort to offer them a scholarly and professional background] (Martín Villar 1979, 4). The remainder of the association's inaugural issue discusses the outcomes of its most recent national conferences, the circulation of the organization's guiding statutes, a brief medical history of hemophilia, and an article on the prospects for youth employment in Spain. In developing these themes, the content of the journal focuses on strategies for disrupting the negative portrayal of hemophilia in popular culture while supplying information and affirmations for young hemophiliacs, who are repeatedly referenced as future leaders and, broadly, the future of Spain. It is an aspirational model which is tilted toward the future, toward the hope of getting somewhere better than the situation they are currently in. As one of the articles concludes: 'Estamos tan cerca y, sin embargo, tan lejos' [We're so close and yet so far] (Martín Villar 1979, 19).

The next few issues of *Nueva Imagen* follow suit, underscoring the social issues and stigmas facing the disease along with its representation in society, and the possibility (or pipe dream, depending on how one might read these articles) of a future cure for hemophilia. In short, issues of futurity dominate these pages, and the association continually attempts to counteract negative representation with images of hemophilic youth and good health. In the second issue, published in the late spring of 1980, the cover directly deploys such a strategy: in a sepia-colored cover image, a young boy stares directly into the camera and at the journal's audience, smiling widely. His sleeves are rolled up, his right arm extended as he uses his left hand to hold a cotton bandage to where he has recently had an injection. Behind him, just out of range of the camera, an adult is seated, writing something down. Above this figure are a few words: '¿Para cuándo la pastilla?' [When will we have the pill?] The appeal to the audience rests on the smiling, cherubic image of this child: why would you want him to suffer further? Although it pins hopes on a (to this day, unavailable) pill that could combat the effects of hemophilia in one's blood and replace the required injections of blood product, the reference to a potential future is coupled with and made dependent on the desire to protect this child and his childhood.

In 1982, shortly before news of HIV/AIDS reached the larger hemophiliac community, family life was once again appealed to with another happy kid and his needles. The cover of the seventh issue of *Nueva Imagen* foregrounds a pre-adolescent boy at a table outdoors. A man, in camouflage and clutching a fishing rod, unloads camping items from a car in the background; further back, a woman in a bright red blouse crouches down, attending to a baby who is seated in the grass and playing with a bright red wheelbarrow. The woman and baby are a cluster of bright red, two drops of blood in the earthy pastoral setting of the campsite. The eye is drawn to them naturally, even though the real activity of the image is the boy in the foreground, who is incongruously injecting himself with plasma product. At his table, one sleeved rolled up and a syringe and tube inserted into his arm, he holds up a cylinder of plasma product and is shown treating himself. Before him on the table are the scattered effects of this treatment—a bandage, packaging, some extra tubing, some cotton wipes—along with a plate and a few cups. The image thus slips between a mundane family excursion to the countryside and the purportedly private act of treatment for hemophilia, and in doing this it seeks to normalize such treatment, blending what is ostensibly a medically private scenario with the familial public. In this manner, *Nueva Imagen* attempts to destabilize illness, challenging what is often the privatized nature of sickness by locating it in the nest of a healthy family, which in turn comes to stand in as a symbol of a healthy nation.

These images serve many functions, as I hope to have made evident: they frame hemophilia as a relatively harmless illness once treated properly, they wrap sickness up into healthy community and family, and they provide a camera-ready face to combat what is often thought of as the ugliness of illness. These are representational strategies, tactics designed to negotiate the experience of liminality from illness. In some ways, they also provide an answer to Butler's question on the language available to the unrecognized; that is, the pre-AIDS era hemophiliac co-opts notions of health and goodness, family and happiness in order to reframe the experience of illness. Butler is quick to note how often this happens, but she also highlights that there are those who would say that any attempt to co-opt the dominant language

> simply culminates in the domestication of the claim. It will end up being an assimilation of the claim; that claim will be contained within the dominant power. That there's no way of entering into using that

> language, misusing it, opening up something through it because no such resistance is possible, no such subversion is possible. (Butler and Rabinow 2001, 40)

She ultimately disagrees with this stance, preferring to focus on the changes made to the language of the dominant once it has been contaminated by the external force of the unrecognized other. Yet there is no attempt at subversion here by the hemophiliac, on the eve of the AIDS epidemic—these are assimilationist policies at work, tactics which seek recognition within a system of institutional gain, rather than an attempt to dismantle the inequalities of such a system. The hemophiliac before AIDS, as *Nueva Imagen* and its sister journals *Fedhemo* and *Hemofilia* show, was concerned with projecting normalcy onto illness, and he was willing to utilize the figures of childhood and futurity to accomplish this goal.

These strategies met resistance as AIDS began to make its impact within the hemophiliac community, and as associations with drug users and homosexuals began to cloud the fantasy of a normative future for hemophiliacs. The type of ideological slip captured in the naming of the 'homophiliac' shows the thinness of whatever vesture of normalcy hemophiliacs had attempted to cover themselves with, alongside the potential that their children could be abducted from them, casualties of the bad associations that plagued them. In effect, the efforts at producing an image of youth that accessed health and happiness proved just as easily infectible by sex, danger, or risk, and in return, hemophiliacs were forced to press further on the figure of the child to offer up a means of exit from a group of risky citizens.

Reporting to their readership in the 1983 issue of *Nueva Imagen*, the editors set a clear outline of the difference between hemophilia and the populations affected by AIDS: 'La prensa ha dedicado especial atención estas últimas fechas a una nueva enfermedad, detectada entre la población homosexual de Nueva York y California. Esta enfermedad [es] normalmente llamada "Plaga Gay" y conocida entre los profesionales de la medicina como AIDS (Síndrome de Deficiencia Inmunológico Adquirida' [The press has dedicated special attention lately to a new illness, detected in the homosexual populations of New York and California. This illness [is] normally called 'Gay Plague' and known among medical professionals as AIDS] (Mendoza García 1983, 2). These are, of course, regrettably familiar tactics: isolating the illness to homosexuals in large urban centers in the United States, underscoring that it is normally called a 'gay plague' while offering up its medical nomenclature with an English acronym. Even the title of the editorial, 'El AIDS', attempts to retain the linguistic foreignness of the illness, keeping it at arm's length.

As it continues by turning to the potential routes of transmission of AIDS, the editorial recurs to medical guidelines, at once cautiously optimistic and wary:

> El riesgo para un afectado de hemofilia por esta enfermedad es mínimo, por el momento. Los expertos del Centro de Control de Atlanta no recomiendan ningún cambio en el uso de productos derivados de la sangre; por lo que no hay ninguna razón para cambiar, de ninguna forma, el tratamiento de hemofilia por infusión. (Mendoza García 1983, 2)[27]

To be clear, the association had few other options at that moment, and it walked a fine line between the threat of non-treatment—which would assuredly cause deaths within its population—and the phantoms of an illness that could be more or less blamed on others.[28]

Nueva Imagen ceased publication after its May 1984 issue, to be replaced a year later by the journal *Hemofilia* (which ran from 1985 to 1988).[29] In its

27 'The risk posed to the hemophiliac by this illness is minimal, for the moment. Experts of the CDC in Atlanta do not recommend any change in the use of products derived from blood; for that reason there is no reason to change, in any way, the treatment of hemophilia by injection.'

28 In this same issue, an interview with the secretary general of the association, Enrique Martínez de Galinsoga, provides a dramatically ironic footnote to its coverage of the emerging AIDS epidemic. Explaining how the association had been fighting for national plasma centers for over two years, Martínez de Galinsoga laments that the current socialist government has been difficult to work with, grimly concluding that the administration has abandoned them (Mendoza García 1983, 3). Galinsoga also discusses the fight to prohibit the uncontrolled dispersal of untested blood products to pharmacies. That is, a testing delay in their dispersal would allow for the retirement of infected batches prior to their distribution, rather than sending out infected blood before its actual status is known. The importance of these continued fights with the reluctant socialist government cannot be understated, as every measure Galinsoga remarks upon here would have undoubtedly limited the spread of HIV/AIDS.

29 After *Hemofilia* ceased publication in 1988, the Spanish Association of Hemophilia did not put out another journal until 1993, when it published the first issue of *Fedhemo* as the Spanish Federation of Hemophilia. The opening editorial is blistering in its accounting for the federation's haphazard publication record: 'Han sido años difíciles, en los que cuando los Hemofílicos habíamos alcanzado el mayor bienestar hasta entonces conocido, se cernió sobre nosotros una infección a la que nosotros habíamos sido ajenos hasta aquel momento, y en la que nunca tuvimos que ver involucrados. Fueron años en los que el desconcierto y desconocimiento de aquella nueva desgracia impidió la realización de otras actividades, que no fueran las destinadas directamente a intentar paliar, en la medida de lo posible, el gravísimo

final issue, *Nueva Imagen* makes one last effort at collapsing innocence and futurity into the figure of the hemophiliac child, divesting itself of the phantom of pathological difference brought about by illness. On its cover, an image of a boy staring forward with his hands in his pockets is shown. The child is drawn in black and white, with the markings of a topographical map filling in the body, lazily contoured lines creating a ripple effect on him. On both sides, his outline has been reproduced three times, each one filled in by alternating colors in blue, purple, and red. The seven figures stand in a V-formation, with the colorless boy in the center. Underneath them, the headline: '¿Distintos? NO, con el plasma de tu sangre' [Different? No, with the plasma from your blood.] The precise meaning of this cover is opaque at best, but it seems to strike at many of the same issues discussed in this chapter. That is, the boy in the center, absent of the color that his faceless shadow-siblings have, both embodies and challenges the notion of difference. He is visibly shown as different by his lack of color and in the wavy markings on his skin and clothes, but his outline provides the shape of the children who stand next to him. The title underneath calls on notions of isolation and difference while also advocating solidarity; the child is a repository for your blood and plasma, waiting to be filled. The altruistic donation of blood—your act of kindness, your extension of healthy citizenship to the recoverable other—will negate his difference, will fill in his lines with color. The end result of this cover strikes at the heart of fears surrounding HIV and AIDS, which is that the infected other is too unlike the healthy citizen; the Hemophiliac Association, however, proved itself adept at utilizing childhood as cultural and social panacea, and it resists being folded into the bad bloodstreams of homosexuals and drug users, who have tainted themselves by their own actions.

Calling forth innocence and futurity in this manner, however, does something queer to the notion of childhood. The kids on the association's magazine covers are too close to blood, handling needles and smiling out at the reader, and dangerously looped into homosexuality by casual linguistic slips. These are children who, unlike those who populate the opening credits of *Más vale prevenir*, are already too close to danger, already too much at risk. How can they be saved? Returning to Kathryn Bond Stockton, we

mal causado' [These have been difficult years, as just when we hemophiliacs had reached a level of wellbeing previously unknown to us, an infection to which we had been unconnected up to that time—and with which we never should have been involved—loomed over us. These were years in which the uncertainty about and ignorance of this new tragedy prevented the fulfillment of any other activities not directly destined to attempt to curb in whatever way possible this most grave harm caused to us] (Federación Española de Hemofilia 1993, 5).

see a similar problematic emerge in pro-family, anti-gay representations of children. Stockton writes that such images exist 'in order to oppose them to each other, fighting the threat of homosexuality under the banner of "what's good for children." Yet by doing so, they make the concept of homosexuality central to the meaning of the children they embrace' (2009, 3). Here, it is not exactly homosexuality (or rather, it is not exclusively homosexuality) that imperils the figure of the child, but the threat of difference, of a fundamental genetic non-normalcy that would place the sick person outside of the constitutive boundaries of the healthy body politic. How do we read the images of children injecting themselves or holding bandages to their arms, existing within the happy family setup even as they are outside of it? Or the child whose body is set apart as different from the outset, whose purpose is to straddle the line between 'you' and the other? Attempting to allay fears of foreignness, illness, or death by employing them to serve on one's behalf taints the figure of the child, forcing him to collude with difference from the outset.

It is difficult to know how transformative representational strategies like these can be, in one way or another. In the years that followed, children with hemophilia were denied access to public playgrounds and schools and were bullied and forced to hide their illness for fear of its then-unknown infectious powers and social stigma. In the face of such immobilizing discrimination—to say nothing of the lack of treatment for AIDS for years to come—any attempt to utilize the figure of the child seems callous. Hasn't the kid been through enough? That potential still calls out, though, to imagine a way in which the child with AIDS might offer a new way of envisioning innocence, sexuality, and illness. Butler's dialogue with Rabinow seems to hold a clue to this potential, as she remarks about engaging with the 'insistent mundaneness' of 'intense dissonance', and allowing it to 'break open to something else, until it becomes unsustainable in some way' (Butler and Rabinow 2001, 45).

Perhaps engaging in this way with such dissonance—in which the figure of the child collides with (what was then) the immanent mortality of AIDS—explodes both concepts. The children happily injecting themselves, then, force us to imagine death, mortality, and blood alongside our conceptualizations of health and nationhood; the difference that *Nueva Imagen* refuses, the image of the boy with your blood in his veins, in fact revives illness and otherness, that weird blur that is produced when your blood becomes his. Even the metaphors of blood that serve as backdrop to these imaginings force queer connections between what is healthy or sick, what the nation is and what it is not. At the onset of the AIDS epidemic, and as it continued, the strategies employed to corral illness either failed or worked depending on who utilized them and when, depending on their attempts to normalize or subvert. But in truth, childhood had already been opened up to the queerness of illness and AIDS, it had already fundamentally shifted its boundaries when the first two brothers succumbed to opportunistic infections. Why else would it need such vigilant protection, such that a father takes on the burden of illness in order to shield his son from its deadly promise? Why else would we need to keep it away from scissors, vacuum cleaners, heights, or from needles, blood, and sex?

CHAPTER THREE

Perverts and Sickos

In a now-infamous exchange on October 15, 1982, between the White House Press Secretary Larry Speakes and reporter Lester Kinsolving, Speakes was asked whether the administration and President Reagan had any response to the growing AIDS epidemic in the United States. At the time of the press briefing, the U.S. death toll had surpassed 800 people. Speakes replied to the question, 'What's A-I-D-S?' Kinsolving answered: 'It's known as the "gay plague".' There were some chuckles around the pressroom at this remark, and Speakes dryly quipped, 'I don't have it, do you?' As he would continue to do every time Kinsolving brought up the epidemic in press briefings throughout subsequent years, Speakes then went on to remark upon the reporter's interest in the topic, openly questioning his sexuality and sending a coded dismissal of both the topic and its source.[1]

A remarkably similar exchange took place in Spain, on an episode of the television program *Fin de siglo* on January 25, 1987. Airing from 1985 to 1987, the show's format consisted of a loose series of interviews around a variety of topics, which were alternated by musical acts. Two participants from this particular episode were especially notable: Rafael Nájera, virologist and leading AIDS expert in Spain at the time, and Juan Barranco, the mayor of Madrid from 1986 to 1989. Over the course of the episode, Nájera answers several questions about the HIV/AIDS epidemic and responds to the quoted statistic of over 100 AIDS-related deaths in Spain to date.[2] The show's host turns to Barranco, who has remained quiet during these exchanges, and

1 Although this exchange has been widely documented, filmmaker Scott Calonico is responsible for unearthing the audio recordings of the press briefing; compiling this and several years of encounters between Kinsolving and Speakes, Calonico created a short documentary, *When AIDS Was Funny*. The documentary debuted on the website for *Vanity Fair*. See Calonico (2015) for more information.

2 As noted throughout this book, tabulations of deaths from AIDS-related causes were both underreported and highly politicized. Any 'official' number given at this time can be assumed to be much underestimated.

says: 'Señor Barranco, no ha intervenido nada en esto del SIDA. Para usted, ¿hay una cuestión del SIDA que te preocupe especialmente, en la que usted tenga interés en particular?' [Mr. Barranco, you haven't made any comments in this discussion about AIDS. For you, is there something about AIDS that especially worries you, something in which you are particularly interested?] After only a brief moment, Barranco answers: 'Bien, yo he propuesto una vacuna' [I've proposed a vaccine.] There are some muffled laughs and murmurs from the audience, who seem both confused and interested. Barranco continues, stating that his vaccine is 'a base de nitratos' [made up of nitrates]. After a pause for comedic effect, he delivers the punchline: 'Pues, "ni trato" con éste, "ni trato" con aquella...' [I 'don't deal' with him, 'I don't deal' with her...] (*Fin de siglo* 1987). The audience, along with the other interviewees at the table, begin to laugh and clap at the joke.

The pivot to humor by Speakes and Barranco is not uncommon in mediated interventions of this sort, particularly when there is little or nothing to say in regard to official policy announcements. Nevertheless, the dismissal of the topic makes patent the lack of seriousness afforded to HIV/AIDS at these politically charged junctures in Spain and the United States. Whether unaware of the epidemic until Kinsolving's query or not, Speakes set aside the seriousness of the outbreak due to the sexual identity of those who were dying from it; Barranco, in a comparable move, quipped that the best 'vaccine' was not to deal with any HIV-positive person at all. Both politicians shrug off the effects of the epidemic by centering their sexual, political, and social identities as normative, which in turn isolates anyone with HIV as aberrant or exceptional. The end result is a policy that is at once social and political, and that keeps the healthy quarantined from the sick.

To television audiences and the larger public (to say nothing of the governments themselves), these exchanges endorsed avoidance of the sick body, along with its containment and isolation into a discrete, exceptional group of the sick. Even in the supposed humor of their political non-policies (a tactic that allows the powerful to pass off their words as 'just a joke' or 'not serious'), Speakes and Barranco reveal their fear of contagion. 'I don't have it, do you?' and 'Pues, ni trato con éste, ni trato con aquella...' are two sides of the same coin, a dismissal of those with HIV as infectious, dangerous, not normal, and in need of monitoring so that they can be identified and studiously avoided. The exclusionary tactic of their humor thus shuts down the pathways that connect communities to each other while controlling and prioritizing certain groups above others.

Such a reactionary stance is nothing new when dealing with illness. In fact, I see the remarks of both men as emerging out of the historical fear of contamination and contagion. This fear in turn reflects common preoccupations with the harm that proximity to the sick body can do and the ways that one's discrete sense of self can be affected through interaction with another. In *Abnormal: Lectures at the Collège de France, 1974–1975* (2003), Foucault claims that such fears originated during the specific quarantine practices of the plague in the eighteenth century—practices which ultimately served to create a disciplinary power that he refers to as 'normalization'. Working from George Canguilheim's *The Normal and the Pathological* (1966), Foucault characterizes normalization as 'an element on the basis of which a certain exercise of power is founded and legitimized' and a political concept that 'brings with it a principle of both qualification and correction' (2003, 50). This is to say that, for Foucault, illness has the capacity to be harnessed as (bio)power over others, a power to be exercised in order to 'correct' and cure the sick. Of course, the exercise of this power in the 'correction' and curing of others—as will be made patent in this chapter—might look nothing like a restorative, healing, or even pleasant process. Foucault continues by noting that 'the norm's function is not to exclude and reject. Rather, it is always linked to a positive technique of intervention and transformation, to a sort of normative project' (2003, 50). As a politically motivated system of power, normalization thus functions by identifying, monitoring, and curing the bad germ (the abnormal cell that threatens the body politic) via its quarantine; in this way, it professes to keep the state healthy and uncontaminated.[3]

Normalization parses individuals from their larger communities in an act of power that colludes with and enforces dominant paradigms of health, sex, and gender. Foucault writes that 'there is a series of fine and constantly observed differences between individuals who are ill and those who are not. It is a question of individualization; the division and subdivision of power extending to the fine grain of individuality' (2003, 46). The meticulous observation of and control over the sick individual[4] thus centers around

3 According to Foucault's analysis, the history of quarantine is long, dating back to the early modern period; in *Abnormal*, however, he specifically highlights the distinction between the sick person's exile from the community (a practice used for lepers, for example) and the vigilant quarantine of the plague-ridden. He further demarcates these two practices as originating and extending certain sociolegal controls over all people by way of control over the sick populace (2003, 44–52).

4 In the category of the 'sick individual', Foucault directs his attentions specifically to the plague (as opposed to the major illness of the seventeenth century, leprosy) and the socializing effects produced in its victims. He does note, however, that the category has a multivalence that has slowly developed over the ensuing centuries, and has resulted in the extension of systems of political and juridical power over the broader categories of sickness and the sick.

the 'question of producing a healthy population' (2003, 46), one that must be policed in order to be kept safe. The state of quarantine (and the quarantine enacted by the state) ultimately produces conflicting political 'dreams', as Foucault refers to them: one that desires release from the law and lawfulness, and the obverse, a fantasy of utter state control in the form of 'an exhaustive sectioning of the population by political power, the capillary ramifications of which constantly reach the grain of individuals themselves, their time, habitat, localization, bodies' (2003, 47). At the height of the AIDS epidemic, the desire for such a deep intervention in political life (such as the segregation and sectioning of the populace in order to maintain safety) became a powerful motivator for the implementation of government practices and mediated messaging in visual culture.

This chapter examines the effects of policing the sick, taking into particular consideration how such 'sickness' is defined—as perverse desires, uncontrollable urges, or physical ills. I examine how certain sexualities in Spain became policed and criminalized through both metaphorical and medical practices, even after their legal decriminalization following the Franco dictatorship. By shifting focus to the works produced in response to the constant policing of sexuality, this chapter offers a counterweight to the studies of dictatorial and democratic practices surrounding queerness and sex. The range of audiovisual cultural products and ephemera produced at this time speaks to the plasticity and nimbleness of feeling sick and offers snapshots of communities struggling to incorporate not only HIV/AIDS but the sense of being deviant, degenerate, or inverted. The ephemera produced by gay collectives like EHGAM (Euskal Heriak Gay Askapen Mugimendua) and regional anti-AIDS committees in Spain emphasize issues such as community engagement, education, safe sex, and resistance to governmental stigma and community pressure; the performance piece 'SIDA da' by Las Pekinesas (1984) uses humor to defuse the queer panic behind the epidemic; while a safe sex comic by Nazario playfully toys with queer desires and sex as a framework for talking about risk and illness. This chapter looks at examples of these responses to pathologization in order to get a sense of being queer and sick in Spain at the time, making the case that from an institutional standpoint, these two things were hardly different.

For Foucault, the incorporation of the sick into the political and social bodies of the state emblematizes the modern production of power, which does not 'act by excluding but rather through a close and analytical inclusion of elements', thereby creating a system of governance and control (2003, 48). The control enacted by the inclusion—not exclusion—of elements of difference represents a power that 'does not act by separating into large confused masses, but by distributing according to differential individualities, a power that is linked not to ignorance but rather to a series of mechanisms that secure the formation, investment, accumulation, and growth of knowledge' (2003, 48). Funneling power in this manner results in the repartitioning of individual bodies into more or less coherent clusters and creates a power system that is easily transferred into a variety of institutions. In this way, institutional (namely legal and medical) governance of the body becomes the process through which the family, sexuality, and identity also come to be governed. The ultimate result is the sustained production of normativity, within which bodies are policed, kept healthy and correct, and differentiated from those so-called abnormal bodies that do not hold to the terms of wellbeing, in whatever form this takes—political, sexual, mental, or physical. Seeing control over sickness as inherent to institutional design (not an accidental byproduct) questions commonly held presumptions about the purely destructive or chaotic forces of illness, holding up instead its immense creational potential; that is, and by underscoring the formation of government through illness and the plague, Foucault defines population and the liberal state as biologically based, emerging out of illness and fears of its contagious properties. This became the chief way that both queerness and illness were corralled and contained in the early years of the HIV/AIDS pandemic in Spain—with only intermittent success, as we will see.

Contagious queerness

Illness has never been exclusively defined on the basis of the physical, although its physicality is precisely what often causes so much primordial dread. Instead, and as I have insisted throughout this book, sickness—and the perception of who is and isn't sick—has a much more profound area of impact, infecting the ways that we think and feel as well as how we negotiate and interact with others. For Foucault, illness is a foundational pillar of the state's biopolitical control over its citizens, one which permits the isolation of who- or whatever is deemed non-normative on both individual and collective levels. The quarantine and control over the sick *and* the healthy thus allow power to be wielded in the name of the moving target of normativity and in alignment with dominant paradigms of what counts as wrong, sick, or queer, in the broadest sense of all three.

Queer[5] individuals throughout history have been linked to illness and difference in a variety of ways, and often painfully and devastatingly so. As

5 I use 'queer' throughout this book as a way to signal a broad range of non-normative sexualities and genders, and as a pointed rejection of the politics that

explored briefly in the introduction, there is a frequently occurring slippage between queerness and illness in the way both are spoken about; whether employed intentionally or not, the semantic slide lays bare the perceptions of both in society. For Diedrich, connecting the two means that there is a bleed, a comingling that suffuses one with the other such that 'illness itself might be understood as queer' (2016, 22). She locates the capaciousness of both terms as inherent to their very definitions, citing one of the *Oxford English Dictionary*'s entries for 'queer': 'not in normal condition; out of sorts; giddy, faint, or ill' (2016, 22). In Spanish, a similar semantic construct occurs in the euphemism 'invertido' [inverted], a slur which was often used during the dictatorship to signify queerness (particularly male). The *Real Academia Española* defines the verb 'invertir' as 'cambiar, sustituyéndolos por sus contrarios, la posición, el orden o el sentido de las cosas' [to change, substituting things by their opposites, position, order, or sense of things] ('Invertir' n.d.). Both 'queer' and 'invertido' highlight deviations from the normal order and shape of the world; in the former, queerness is bent and out of normal condition, and in the latter queerness inverts order and the sense of normalcy. What is normal is thus rendered in formal, figurative terms, which the queer bends and inverts.

Illness, similarly, is often seen and defined as an abnormal state of the mind and body, the corruption of the purportedly natural state of things. If these two can be folded in on each other—and from these foundational similarities, I believe they can—then the biopolitical control exercised over illness has much deeper and more far-reaching power than previously imagined, as it will necessarily include types of queerness that are most often seen as products of mental infirmity or disorder. Containing illness becomes another way to contain queerness, in the very real ways that these two have been collapsed into each other across a variety of state apparatuses. For that reason (and though the particularities of anti-queer legal discrimination in Spain are fairly well known), it might be useful here to gloss some of the most infamously homophobic legislation produced during the early years of AIDS in Spain. By this, I want to further highlight

only paints a specific type of person (i.e., white, gay, cisgender) as the AIDS victim *par excellence*. Though queer originated as a slur against LGBTQ communities, its academic use and reappropriation began in the early 1990s with texts by Teresa de Lauretis (1991) and Annamarie Jagose (1996), to name only two of many. In Spain, 'queer' did not appear in academic use until the early 2000s, broadly speaking, in theorists like David Córdoba, Javier Sáez, and Paco Vidarte (2005), who worked to adapt its use to a Spanish context. For a detailed contextualization of the debates that emerged from Córdoba et al.'s employment of the term in the early 2000s, see Epps (2009).

how illness and queerness have long been cast together, and how the legal repression and social stigmatization of queerness has regulated perceptions and performances of masculinity and femininity.

It should be noted that the guiding ethos of the Franco dictatorship's misogyny and homophobia has been scrutinized and criticized in a number of cross-disciplinary studies: Oscar Guasch's sociologically based work on homosexuality in society, particularly *La sociedad rosa* (1994); a great number of Paul Julian Smith's writings, including *Vision Machines: Cinema, Literature, and Sexuality in Spain and Cuba, 1983–93* (1996) and *Television in Spain: From Franco to Almodóvar* (2006); Alberto Mira's *De Sodoma a Chueca* (2004), which covers very nearly the entirety of gay history in Spain; Gema Pérez-Sánchez's *Queer Transitions in Contemporary Spanish Culture* (2007), which is quoted at length in this chapter and uses literary works to examine the specific reactions to and representations of legal and political repression of queerness; Alejandro Melero's visual studies on representations of lesbians and gays in film in *Placeres ocultos: Gays y lesbianas en el cine español de la Transición* (2010) and *Violetas de España: Gays y lesbianas en el cine de Franco* (2017); David Vilaseca's *Queer Events: Post-deconstructive Subjectivities in Spanish Writing and Film, 1960s to 1990s* (2010); and Chris Perriam's *Spanish Queer Cinema* (2013). This necessarily incomplete list of works—which only gestures toward the scope of LGBTQ and queer studies in Spain over the past couple of decades—demonstrates the ample intellectual effort that has been applied to understanding how social and legal repression has affected queer cultures in Spain.

Notably, many of these projects attempt to understand repression through the regime's rigid stratification of masculinity and femininity. Pérez-Sánchez, for example, writes that 'Francoist political, religious, social, and cultural institutions attempted to reconstruct a dominant Spanish identity predicated on nineteenth-century gender roles' (2007, 21). Through this, she concludes that Francoism's focus on containing homosexuality was related to

> a two-fold sense of the threat of feminization: on the one hand, the general population must have felt as if it were located in a passive, feminine position, but on the other hand, the Francoist regime itself occupied a marginalized, subservient position with respect to the rest of the Western world. (2007, 22)

The threat posed by such feminization, according to Pérez-Sánchez, resulted in the dictatorship's attempts to 'rigidly [fix] proper gender roles and heterosexual practices' among 'men who did not seem acceptably masculine, who were perceived—from a simplistic, heterosexist view—to allow themselves to be sodomized, that is, who willingly embraced what was considered the passive, feminine position' (2007, 22). Pérez-Sánchez is right to point to the fixed ideals of the dictatorship as hyper-focused on the 'correct' performance of masculinity and femininity, according to its narrowly informed framework. But is domination always suffered passively or by those in a passive (and therefore feminized) position? Is authority only ever enacted through masculinized aggression?[6] Instead of reducing the complicated performances of gender in such a way, we might instead look to the biopolitical control over queerness-as-illness, and the quarantine of illness as a queer state of the body and as means of dominance.[7] These approaches are far from mutually exclusive, as control over conceptualizations of wellness is intimately tied to the governance of normative gender roles and sexual identities. Thus, by widening the scope of what counts as dictatorial control—and control over the health of the body was clearly enacted in the dictatorship—we can understand how the regime's motivations were steeped in categorical wellness and the ways in which bodies were contained and quarantined, normalized and managed according to dominant ideals of social and national health.

In his chapter of the edited collection *El homosexual ante la sociedad enferma*, Armand de Fluvià writes about the legal repression of homosexuals in Spain over the centuries, moving from the horrific stake burnings of the fifteenth century to the more lax laws of the Second Republic and back to the rigid criminalization of the Franco dictatorship. He lingers longest, however,

6 By way of example: in 'Resemanticising Feminine Surrender: Cross-gender Identifications in the Writings of Spanish Female Fascist Activists' (2002), Jo Labanyi takes apart the dominant perception of wholesale female submission during the dictatorship, particularly within the ranks of the fascist female organization Sección Feminina. Reading against the models that equate fascist femininity with subjugation, Labanyi argues for a more nuanced perception of women's work in the Francoist period, one that afforded (limited) freedoms and the exercise of agency within a heavily codified system of gender.

7 To be clear, the dictatorship was most certainly fixated on reproducing normative gender roles. The tendency to highlight this fixation may ironically be responsible in part for the continued critical focus on gay men and their (perceived lack of) masculinity. As is the case with the law during the dictatorship, there appears to be a lacuna of sorts when it comes to imagining homosexuality and queerness beyond men who have sex with men. For an analysis of lesbian invisibility in times of queer criminalization, see Vila Núñez (1999) and Chapter 2 of Pérez-Sánchez's *Queer Transitions in Contemporary Spanish Culture* (2007); for a brief overview of the legal status of the transgender community during and after the dictatorship, see Araneta and Fernández Garrido (2016).

on the two best-known dictatorial laws that criminalized homosexuality: the Ley de Vagos y Maleantes, which was issued in 1933 and modified in 1954 to specifically include homosexuality,[8] and the Ley de Peligrosidad y Rehabilitación Social, issued in 1970. Punishments for transgressing these laws varied, including internment in so-called 're-education' camps, jail sentences, and/or temporary expulsion or permanent exile from certain places and spaces as designated by the authorities (de Fluvià 1978b, 91–92).

The 1933 version of the Ley de Vagos y Maleantes crafted a list of social undesirables (in the language of the time: ruffians, pimps, beggars, the mentally ill, and the handicapped, among a few others) and articulated the control that the government should have over them. Describing the punishment applied to this motley group of alleged deviants, Pérez-Sánchez notes how the early version of this law 'envisions a future' for them 'as productive, content farmers' via their relocation to the state's agricultural work camps, which would 'force them to become useful members of society, thus reforming their evil ways through hard labor—a measure that would serve the added function of benefiting capitalistic society at large' (2007, 29). This happy agrarian future, however, was only possible for the type of deviance that fell within a specific set of boundaries. The 1954 revision to the law that formally brought homosexuality under its scope forced the state to contend with the lines between containable and incorrigible deviance, leading perhaps to the notion that rehabilitation might not be possible for homosexuals, despite the state's best punitive efforts. This revision further introduced specific procedures applying to homosexuals (namely, internment in the aforementioned work/re-education camps) that were enacted in order to keep gay men separate from other criminals. These measures effectively allowed for 'a parallel series of solutions for homosexuals that are separate and different from those provided for the other dangerous subjects' (Pérez-Sánchez 2007, 28), the function of which, as Juan Vicente Aliaga describes, was to 'impedir que se propagasen y extendieran los actos de coyunda homosexual, al parecer contagiosos: una de las típicas, y más frecuentes, paranoias de la institución heterosexista' [prevent the spread and extension of the apparently contagious act of homosexual coupling: one of the typical, and most frequent, paranoias of the heterosexist institution] (Aliaga and Cortés 1997, 28). Both Pérez-Sánchez and Aliaga point directly to the fear behind this particular revision of the

8 Though the law was formally amended in 1954 to include homosexuality, state records indicate that homosexuals were being tried under the Ley de Vagos y Maleantes at least a decade prior to its official revision. See Olmeda (2004) and Heredia Urzáiz (2009).

law—that of contagious queerness, 'a particularly infectious brand of dangerousness' (Pérez-Sánchez 2007, 28–29) that inspires paranoia, gay panic, and the need for quarantine.

The 1970 Ley de Peligrosidad y Rehabilitación Social, in contrast, directly addressed homosexuality from the outset,[9] and in so doing strengthened further the divide between healthy normalcy (read: heterosexuality) and sick queerness. One of the more notable differences between this law and its predecessor, as Jordi Petit notes, was that 'desde el punto de vista jurídico se trataba de una ley peculiar que no perseguía tanto la comisión de actos "peligrosos", sino a los sujetos de los mismos, los practicaren o no en el momento de su detención' [From a legal point of view, it was a peculiar law that did not so much pursue the committing of 'dangerous' acts, but rather the subjects of these, whether or not they were performing them at the time of their arrest] (2003, 27). Following this logic, it becomes clear that the branding of homosexuals as dangerous—rather than the supposed homosexual acts that they committed, whatever these might be—thus reimagined danger and lawlessness themselves as characteristics inherent to queer identities. Citing the law directly, Armand de Fluvià observes how:

> Los sujetos incluidos dentro de la ley son juzgados con criterios subjetivos, ya que el texto legal habla de quienes hayan 'voluntariamente o no podido quedar marginados de una vida ordenada y normal' ... De esta forma, se establecen unos arquetipos de sujetos y unos módulos de comportamiento 'ordenados' y 'normales': los que no alteren las relaciones de dominación; arquetipos de sujetos y módulos de comportamiento pretendidamente 'pacíficos', que no alteren la vida social en un modo de producción no precisamente pacífico. Los sujetos que no se incluyan dentro de estos arquetipos y módulos 'ordenados

9 Llamas and Vila critique the auspicious date of this law, particularly in contrast with a growing global movement calling for an increase in protections and rights for the LGBTQ community: 'Un año después de que tenga lugar en Nueva York la Revuelta de Stonewall (y de que empiece a surgir un movimiento reivindicativo en el mundo occidental), se sustituye la Ley de Vagos y Maleantes por una nueva ley que pretendía ser más eficaz y que mostraba hasta qué punto la realidad de lesbianas y gays estaba alejada de los procesos que estaban cohesionando los movimientos de liberación en otros lugares.' [A year after the Stonewall riots took place in New York (and a protest movement began to emerge in the Western world), the Ley de Vagos y Maleantes was replaced by a new law that was intended to be more effective and that showed to what extent the reality of lesbians and gays was removed from the events that were forming liberation movements in other places] (1994, 193).

> y normales' serán susceptibles de ser clasificados como 'peligros sociales'. (1978b, 89–90)[10]

De Fluvià astutely critiques the law's recurrence to normalcy and order, terms that are treated as synonyms and that prize the perception of a natural order that is exclusively defined by the dominant paradigm. Under the guise of 'order', as de Fluvià suggests, the law reinforces its ability to classify what constitutes an abnormal life and sets it up as that which fails to obey the logic of governing cultural norms. The haziness of the law's definitions serves to shore up its enforceability, even as it reveals its utter reliance on an internal sense of whose lives are normal, logical, ordered, and correct.

Both Spanish laws cast queerness as an infectious social illness, and both insinuate that homosexuality is an infirmity that adheres to the individual regardless of recent actions or sexual partners. This is made manifest in the original design of the laws themselves, as when Mariano Ruiz-Funes, co-author of the Ley de Vagos y Maleantes, opined that 'el conceder una gracia colectiva a los peligrosos equivaldría a ignorar la verdadera naturaleza de la peligrosidad. Sería algo tan extraño como afirmar que se puede perdonar al enfermo su enfermedad' [to grant a collective pardon to dangerous people would be to ignore the true nature of dangerousness. It would be something as strange as affirming that the sick person can be forgiven his illness] (qtd. in Monferrer Tomás 2003, 186). Monferrer Tomás, underscoring the language used by Ruiz-Funes, points out that these laws defined the dangerous individual as one who cannot be pardoned but cured; for that reason, 'en prevención del contagio, se considerará necesario aislarlos del cuerpo social, reeducar, y reintegrar únicamente cuando se considere que estén curados' [in prevention of contagion, it will be considered necessary to isolate them from the social body, re-educate, and reintegrate them only when it is considered that they are cured] (2003, 186). But what might such a 'cure' actually look like, when doer and deed are so tightly linked? Or to push this thought

10 'The subjects included within the law are judged with subjective criteria, since the legal text speaks of those who have "whether voluntarily or not remained outside the bounds of an orderly and normal life" ... In this way, there are established archetypes of subjects and modes of "orderly" and "normal" behavior: those that do not alter relationships of domination; archetypes of subjects and modules of behavior that are supposedly "peaceful", that do not alter social life in a mode of production that is not precisely peaceful. Subjects that are not included within these "ordered and normal" archetypes and modes will be susceptible to being classified as "social dangers".'

further, how would one ever go about separating sickness from queerness, when the laws designed to control them function only on the basis of their coexistence?

Such tight control over queerness cannot be maintained without a highly organized relationship between medical and legal norms and institutions. That is, the criminalization of certain physical and mental pathologies, like the pathologizing of certain criminals, binds both groups to an idealized vision of wellbeing that prizes certain social and political definitions of normalcy. Moreover, the criminalization of queerness under Franco was intimately tied to—and justified through—its pathologization by the dominant medical structures of the time. In much of the world, and particularly in Europe, this fell to the World Health Organization (WHO) via the United Nations. Spain joined the WHO in 1951, after it was initially denied access to the United Nations as a result of its support of the Axis powers during the Second World War. Consequently, with the exception of the original Ley de Vagos y Maleantes (which was promulgated during the Second Republic and, as mentioned, notably did not include homosexuality in its original incarnation), all of its homophobic regulations were written under the aegis of medically sanctioned discrimination.[11] Given the weight afforded to conservative Catholic doctrine during the dictatorship (and for centuries prior), the discrimination against homosexuality prior to the introduction of the WHO guidelines is wholly unsurprising; it is nonetheless revealing that the 1951 integration into the WHO paved the way for the explicit naming and inclusion of homosexuality into existing law. In this manner, the use of medicine to shore up discriminatory practices and

11 Homosexuality was formally de-pathologized in the United States in 1973, when the American Psychiatric Association removed it from the second edition of the DSM (Diagnostic and Statistical Manual); in practice, however, it was merely replaced (and re-pathologized) by a new diagnosis of queerness called 'sexual orientation disturbance' in 1973, which was in turn replaced by the diagnosis of 'ego-dystonic homosexuality' in 1980. It was not until 1987 that homosexuality was fully de-pathologized. The competing guidelines of the WHO's International Statistical Classification of Diseases and Related Health Problems (ICD) have been revised at a much slower pace and with very uneven adoption by its member countries. For that reason, homosexuality was removed from the ICD in 1990 but still remained in the formulation of 'ego-dystonic sexual orientation' up to 2019. The newest version of the ICD, version 11, removed ego-dystonic sexual orientation from its list of disorders after a lengthy series of debates and field tests that began in 2007 and were finally approved in 2019. The ICD-11 went into effect in January 2022 and, though it was approved by all members, is likely to be subject to the same unevenness of member adoption. See Drescher (2015) and the World Health Organization (2018) for more.

moral beliefs allows for discrimination against queerness to be reified, underpinned by the purported neutrality of science and law.

This is but a brief summary of how these two laws—alongside the legal and medical institutions that authored them—wielded blunt punitive power over the LGBTQ community in Spain. As a result of this tight control, the state (in both its dictatorial and democratic iterations) crafted a dominant paradigm that equated heterosexuality with health and framed the queer as its inverse, an infectious germ requiring quarantine and containment. Consequently, to be queer was to be sick; to feel queer attachments was to feel such sickness at work, to feel the pull of your contagious, viral sexuality. The stories, ephemera, and actions that emerged from this long period of time thus document an imposed sense of isolation and fear of authoritative punishment. They also demonstrate ways of imagining oneself outside of the quarantine chamber and into spaces that offered freedom of movement from within and without illness.

'SIDA DA'

As we will see, action and resistance against a medico-social system of ill identities can take many forms. One specific example has been documented by members of the archival research group 'Equipo: re' (Aimar Arriola, Nancy Garín, and Linda Valdés), which traces the connections between performance, activism, and the AIDS archives in Spain and Chile. Collaborating closely with Miguel Benlloch, a Spanish performance artist and activist, the group has chronicled a 1984 performance piece on AIDS featuring Las Pekinesas, of which Benlloch was a member with Tomás Navarro and Rafael Villegas. Arriola and Garín describe the performance, titled 'SIDA da', as taking place 'en el sótano de un bar, el Planta Baja, epicentro de la contra-cultura en la ciudad de Granada desde primeros de los 80, co-fundado por Miguel' [in the basement of a bar, the Ground Floor, the epicenter of counterculture in the city of Granada since the early 1980s, co-founded by Miguel] (2014, n.p.). By tying the locale to the counterculture of the 1980s in Spain (a reference that also links the bar to a broader series of countercultural movements in Spain and, in particular, to the Madrid-based *Movida*) and by positioning Benlloch's centrality to these, Arriola and Garín piece together a history that links activism, counterculture, and AIDS as concurrent and interdependent. Such a description is significant, particularly given the manner in which the countercultural movements in Spain in the 1980s are often cast as apolitical and apathetic anti-movements.

In the performance, the three members of Las Pekinesas stood in front of their audience in masks that covered the top halves of their faces. One by one and in rotation, amid audience laughs and performance gaffes, the group recited a series of puns on the word 'SIDA' [AIDS].

> Sida la flecha. / Suma y sida. / Sida del Vaticano. / Sida Calatayud. / Sida París papá, pregunta por los apaches. / Quien va a Sevilla perdió su sida. / Sida y diseño. / Juan Sida. / Planta sida. / Ronald Sida. / Sida Iribarne. / Sida Serra. / Sida Heyworth. / Sida de Fürstenberg. / Zara Sida. / Homisida. / Parrisida. / Regic-sida. / Hirosida mon amour. / Roma, sida aperta. / Con sida y a lo loco. / Cásida de las palomas oscuras. / Cásida del amor y la muerte. / Cásida de la mano imposible. / Sida. (Benlloch, Navarro, and Villegas 1984)

Las Pekinesas recited and read their lines, passing a microphone back and forth over a morose, operatic soundtrack with a steady beat. At one point, one member of the trio forgot his lines, laughingly whispered '¿Cuál era el mío?' [Which was mine?], and looked down at his crib sheet for a reminder. The performers laughed throughout the performance, and the audience laughed with them, acknowledging the playful interchange between the original words and phrases and their satirization. In this manner 'suma y sigue', an idiom meaning 'a great deal' or 'one after another', becomes 'suma y sida', which compounds the sense of AIDS as unstoppable, waves and waves of bodies multiplying and collecting; 'quien va a Sevilla, pierde su silla', another idiom that references the loss of one's possessions after having momentarily abandoned them, is repurposed as 'quien va a Sevilla, perdió su SIDA', a somewhat nonsensical phrase that suggests that one could be cured of AIDS by visiting Seville. Other lines repurpose famous poems, songs, or films, such as 'Si vas a París, Papá', a 1979 song by Los Parchis (reimagined here as 'Sida París, papá...'), 'Con Sida y a lo loco' (*Con faldas y a lo loco / Some Like it Hot*, Billy Wilder, 1979), 'Hirosida, mon amour' (*Hiroshima, mon amour*, Alain Resnais, 1960), 'Roma, Sida aperta' (*Roma città aperta / Rome, Open City*, Roberto Rossellini, 1945) and two poems by Federico García Lorca. Another set of puns reference noted (or notorious) public figures, like Ronald Reagan (Ronald Sida), Manuel Fraga Iribarne (Sida Iribarne), Richard Serra, and Rita Hayworth. Finally, a set of words plays with homophony, referencing homicide, parricide, and regicide.

The richness of the auditory interplay between 'sida' and the cultural figures, events, and works referenced in the piece is at once compelling, overwhelming, and immanently tongue-in-cheek; the textual wordplay, similarly, is alternately poignant and nonsensical, a critique of cultural and political institutions and a whimsical sonic game. Some of the references implicate figures and texts with deep (and at times painful) connections to queerness or HIV/AIDS, as when they allude to Fraga, Reagan, Serra, and Lorca. In other phrases, the transformation of song title or idiom holds out an affecting portrayal of illness, as I noted earlier with 'suma y sida'. 'Con Sida y a lo loco' [With AIDS, and wildly], to offer another example, is a humorous reference to a film with well-established queer resonances that also coins a phrase evoking a particular feeling of having illness, a frenetic sense of being sick. Such affective and affecting moments seem to casually blossom in the midst of the piece's cacophony of repetitive sounds—not only through the continual pun of 'sida' but in the accompanying musical soundtrack. These pockets of affective significance are fleeting, however, which is to say that the connection between the puns and AIDS is often tenuous, nonexistent, or so immensely personal that its immediate meaning is obscured.

As one of the earliest surviving works of visual culture in Spain that deal with the epidemic, 'SIDA da' verbalizes what it means to feel sick, in the expansive sense that I offered in the introduction; that is, it formulates a playfully queer structure of feeling with a strategy for coping and survival that is both a failure and a success of meaning, an act that creates connective links and disruptions with its audience. 'SIDA da' expresses what it feels like to be queer and sick, but it does so in ways we can only partially understand. It doesn't make sense, but then it does. It struggles with language, it forgets its lines. It tries to tell the story of an event that is still in the process of unfolding, and as such it teeters on the 'very edge of semantic availability' (Williams 2009, 134), as structures of feeling do.

In the introduction, I described these sorts of moments—in which emergent linguistic formations, groups, friendships, or meanings are produced in the queer experience of feeling sick—as formational elements of the narratives that converged around AIDS and Spain at this time. As suggested by the linkage that Arriola and Gardín make between Benlloch's activist performance art and his participation in the countercultural movements of the 1980s, the narratives that came out of the epidemic were neither simple nor created in isolation. That is, such stories react to and subvert politics even as they reveal new formulations of sexual identities and wholesale rewrites of the dominant discourses that have solidified around recent Spanish history; just as frequently, they fall apart in pain, are unable to meaningfully convey a message to an audience, or retreat into silence. This slide between failure and success crafts a sort of politics that does not always function on political or social gain but on survival and coping, a management of the everyday ups-and-downs of living through an ongoing (health) crisis. The invocation of humor in 'SIDA da', even—and particularly—when it fails or falls a little flat with nonsense, is therefore able to challenge the words and meanings that have been used by the state to corral the LGBTQ community into submission. By parsing and deconstructing the phonemes that produce the word 'sida', dizzyingly reproduced so often that the word barely seems to stand on its own by the end of the performance, Las Pekinesas offer up a mercurial vision of what illness (and therefore queerness) is. That this did not stop the medicalization of queerness or the stigmatization of AIDS and people with HIV is almost inconsequential, or is at least less consequential than the interruption of this flow of biopower, which in turn disrupts the discursive control of meaning that has been taken up as the exclusive purview of the state. By exploding the semantics of AIDS, emptying the signifier of its pain and filling it with queer meaning and nonsense, Las Pekinesas question the state's dominance over linguistic value and signification.

This reading of 'SIDA da' shares some affinities with what Arriola and Garín have described as 'otras formas de lo político', a strategy of resistance which they use to 'designar un conjunto amplio de estrategias críticas de producción visual y performativa desarrolladas en oposición a las políticas de represión de la dictadura y la transición' [designate a broad set of critical strategies for visual and performative production developed in opposition to the repressive policies of the dictatorship and the Transition] (2014, n.p.). For Arriola and Garín, these other ways of doing politics are intimately connected to the corporeality of the body and playfulness.[12] Though the authors only offer an outline of how such forms of politics might emerge, what shape they take, and how they confront dominant paradigms, they are right to point to the potential of corporeality and the body to disrupt and pick apart the institutional control over meaning. In this book, I have worked to take up their initial thoughts, thinking through illness, loss, and other negative corporealities. In so doing, I see the day-to-day gestures, performances, and movements that accompany living with HIV/AIDS as strategies of resistance and coping, failing and surviving, and toggling between success and failure.

Sex in action

In exposing the connective tissue between institutional discourse and the criminalization of queerness, this book underscores the fundamental connections between queerness and AIDS. These connections are pointedly *not* those that were made in the early years of the epidemic, which were the

12 For more on the queer politics that Benlloch's work creates and imagines, see Jesús Alcaide's observations in 'Sujeto brillante desidentificado' (2020).

simplistic and outmoded associations of sex between men and the belief in a hazard-ridden risk group. Instead, I see the links between queerness and AIDS as the bending, shifting, and weirding pressures enacted on the self that produce sensations of isolation, unease, and pain. These sensations—in which one feels sick, out of sorts in the body, and contained—erupt wildly, politically, and sometimes irrationally, coalescing into a form of body politics that is something akin to what Arriola and Garín have also gestured toward. Such emergent body politics—and the concurrent structures of feeling that they enact—formed the makeup of LGBTQ activism in Spain in the latter half of the twentieth century, which was born out of the techniques of normalization, containment, and medicalization impressed upon the queer communities of Spain during this period.

Though pockets of gay resistance certainly bubbled up in Spain in the years prior to the 1970s,[13] the Ley de Peligrosidad y Rehabilitación Social (LPRS) served as a catalyst for queer activism's earnest rise. According to Armand de Fluvià, one of the pioneers of gay activism in Spain, resistance to the LPRS on the part of the LGBTQ communities and their allies ushered in a wave of gay liberation movements that began in Catalonia and spread through Spain (1978a, 151). Beginning slowly but energetically, de Fluvià and Francesc Francino (under the pseudonyms Roger de Gaimon and Mir Bellgai, respectively) wrote letters to politicians and gay organizations in other countries in opposition to the LPRS. The political ire and pressure generated by Gaimon and Bellgai's protest letters resulted in a minor but consequential shift in the law's language to solely apply to those who committed 'homosexual acts', rather than homosexuals writ large.[14] Buoyed by this political victory, the two brought together a small, clandestine group with the intent to author a monthly publication. This, *Agrupación Homófila para la Igualdad Sexual* (*AGHOIS*), was first published in 1972 and eventually

13 I am taking cues from de Fluvià's writing on one of the earliest (and to his knowledge, only) queer public demonstrations in Spain, which occurred in 1934. De Fluvià cites a passage from Jean Genet's *The Thief's Journal*, which recounts a group of around 30 queer people marching through the streets of Barcelona and toward a bombed-out public urinal. The group, called 'Las Carolinas', carried bouquets of red roses tied with a black ribbon as a sort of mourning for the loss of this public site of queer desire and cruising (de Fluvià 1978a, 149–51). This story is also briefly recounted in Llamas and Vila (1994).

14 The significance of this victory is clear and contributed to the political momentum of the work being done by Francino/Bellgai and de Fluvià/de Gaimon. It should nonetheless be sobered somewhat by the formal practices and punishments of the law, which continued to exceptionalize homosexuality by keeping gay male prisoners separate and apart from others prosecuted under the LPRS, as discussed earlier in the chapter.

led to the formal establishment of the Movimiento Español de Liberación Homosexual (MELH). As a group, MELH had two principal objectives, according to de Fluvià: 'concienciar a los homosexuales para reivindicar sus derechos y conseguir la aceptación y reconocimiento de los mismos por parte de la sociedad' [to raise awareness in homosexuals in order to demand their rights and to obtain acceptance and recognition of the same within society] (1978a, 153). In addition to weekly meetings in Barcelona, the writing and distribution of its publications, and participation in European activism, a (by all accounts, ephemeral) chapter of MELH in Madrid was also formed at this time. In late 1975, the group shifted political tactics as the Franco dictatorship waned with his ill-health. According to Llamas and Vila, this shift was also produced 'en línea con la evolución ideológica que se produce tanto en su propio seno como en el conjunto de los movimientos sociales antifranquistas' [in line with the ideological evolution being produced from within the group as it was in anti-Francoist social movements] (Llamas and Vila 1994, 197). Rechristened as Front d'Alliberament Gai de Catalunya (FAGC), the group took its place with a number of other LGBTQ groups forming across Spain[15] in demanding sexual liberation and social liberties for queer Spaniards. The more combative stance of FAGC—which published its objectives in a 'manifesto' framed in bellicose language—began a more publicly visible era for queer politics, so much so that Armand de Fluvià considered the group's *Manifest* 'el primer análisis político de la cuestión homosexual hecho en el Estado español' [the first political analysis of the homosexual question made in the Spanish state] (1978a, 157). For de Fluvià, this manifesto imagined itself as the 'base para una definitiva elaboración de la teoría de la liberación sexual' [foundation for a definitive elaboration of the theory of sexual liberation] (1978a, 157). Monferrer Tomás notes in agreement that 'a partir de ese momento los temas planteados van a quedar abiertos a debate dentro de la sociedad española, obligando a posicionarse con respecto a ellos a las diferentes instancias de control social, a los actores

15 López Romo describes the seemingly sudden abundance of queer groups in the first few months of 1977 and provides a list of a number of these: 'Nacieron la Unión Democrática Homosexual de Málaga; el Movimiento Homosexual Aragonés (Zaragoza); el Frente de Liberación Homosexual Gallego (Santiago de Compostela); EHGAM (Bilbao); el Frente Homosexual de Acción Revolucionaria, espejo de su homónimo francés; la Agrupación Mercurio y el Movimiento Democrático Homosexual. Estas tres últimas organizaciones coexistieron en Madrid, pero tuvieron una vida más bien efímera. Durante 1978 se fundó el Frente de Liberación Homosexual de Castilla (FLHOC), colectivo que las sucedería. En marzo del 77 también surgió una escisión del FAGC, la llamada Coordinadora de Collectius per l'Alliberament Gai' (López Romo 2008, 52).

sociales relevantes y a la opinión pública' [from this moment on, the ideas proposed (by the Manifesto) remain open to debate in Spanish society, requiring relevant social actors and public opinion to adopt a stance to different instances of social control] (2003, 192–93).

The Front d'Alliberament Gai de Catalunya's struggle for LGBTQ rights was intentionally linked to that of other marginalized groups, and FAGC counted on the 'participación de casi todos los partidos y organizaciones de clase y movimientos marginales y radicales' [participation of almost all parties and organizations related to class and radical marginal movements] (de Fluvià 1978a, 158). This is not only an indication of the more progressive turn of national politics in the wake of the dictator's death, but also of the interconnected sense of struggle that united marginalized political voices in Spain. By tying its fight to the particularly homophobic measures of the Ley de Peligrosidad y Rehabilitación Social, queer activism was able to articulate itself in alignment with a host of other 'deviant' bodies and groups. Its political platform, which according to de Fluvià was 'la base para las plataformas de todos los movimientos de liberación gai del estado español' [the foundation for the platforms of all gay liberation movements in the Spanish state] (1978a, 158), included statements that advocated for the rights of sex workers, equality for women, increased access to sex education, and amnesty for political prisoners (as they considered those who had been incarcerated under the LPRS).[16]

The scale of the task was not lost on activists such as de Fluvià, who were faced with the 'double marginalization' of being not only sexually but politically deviant in the eyes of the state (Pérez-Sánchez 2007, 32). Citing a letter between de Fluvià and an activist counterpart in the United States, Pérez-Sánchez notes how queer activists were stuck 'with the triple task of having to raise consciousness among closeted gays and lesbians and beginning a productive dialogue with progressive heterosexuals while outmaneuvering censorship' (2007, 32), which in de Fluvià's own words was a 'huge and very unrewarding' task (qtd in Pérez-Sánchez 2007, 32). In some ways, it was an uphill battle, as even noted progressives—theoretically, the allies—couched their discussions of homosexuality in the terminology of infirmity. The list of these is lengthy, as López Romo elucidates: Enrique Tierno Galván, beloved progressive mayor of Madrid from 1979 to 1986, referred to queers as 'desviados' [deviants] who needed correction and comprehension, and whose 'relaciones insanas fomentadas dentro del sistema capitalista' [unhealthy relationships encouraged by the capitalist system] existed because of a lack of timely psychiatric treatment (qtd in López

16 See de Fluvià (1978a, 158–61) for the full text of the FAGC manifesto.

Romo 2008, 58–59); Manuel Guedán, member of the Central Committee of the Workers' Revolutionary Organization, referred to homosexuality as an abnormality, alteration of sexuality, and an educational, psychological, or physical deformation (López Romo 2008, 58); Marta Ferrusola, wife of famed president of the Generalitat Jordi Pujol, confessed to not understanding whether homosexuality was 'una tara, un vicio, un defecto o la suma de todo' [a defect, a vice, a flaw or a combination of all three] (qtd in Petit 2003, 96); and others insisted on the broad debility or weakness that queerness demonstrated in the individual and encouraged in society.

These perceptions are wholly indicative of a certain way of thinking that I have worked to highlight over the course of this chapter, which imagines the queer as sick, aberrant, and infirm. I have focused on one of the germs of queer abnormality—the state's regulatory biopolitical practices that determine the health and wellbeing of its citizenry—but the fullness of this notion is sustained powerfully in many ways and with real and damning outcomes for LGBTQ people. Such a multipronged correlation between queerness and illness is one of the through lines of this book. The shoring up of the queer body along the lines of sickness and abnormality may be ultimately regulated by the state, as Foucault has written, but queerness-as-infirmity is not exclusively maintained by state apparatuses or institutions; in fact, there must be some belief in the inherent rightness or veracity of the system in order for it to be so pervasive, as seen in everything from theoretically cooperative social justice organizations to medical professionals and practices.

The histories of LGBTQ activism that lead to the early 1980s, then, can be read along this line—as a battle against the damaging notion that perennially links queers to infirmity. The fight against the LPRS, which is seen to have been the catalyst for modern queer activism in Spain, was one that sought to decouple queerness from abnormality. The *Manifest* put forth by the FAGC, in a similar fashion, forcefully looked to tear down systems of governance that impose measures on the physicality of queer bodies. It is unsurprising, then, that FAGC's broadly progressive stances highlighted the materiality of the body in tandem with the state's unfettered access to those bodies it deemed abnormal or deviant. By way of its manifesto, the group condemned the restriction of heterosexual women and queer folk to certain physical and social spaces, the exile and displacement of queers to specified centers or camps, the chemical regulation of bodies via lack of contraceptives and electroshock treatment/torture, and the legalized restrictions that prohibited the sexual contact of certain bodies. Their *Manifest* took further aim at the explicit psychological, medical, and legal ties that tethered queerness to illness, urging 'NO CONSIDERACIÓN de la homosexualidad como una enfermedad, tanto en la enseñanza como en la práctica médica y psicológica y, en consecuencia, prohibición explícita de aplicar terapias aversivas y todo tipo de tratamiento que tienda a cambiar la conducta sexual' [NO CONSIDERATION of homosexuality as an illness, either in medical and psychological practice or education, and consequently, the explicit prohibition of conversion therapies and any type of treatment that offers to change sexual conduct] (de Fluvià 1978a, 158–61).

Hence, the body—not only as concept but in its actual physicality—has long been an integral concern of queer resistance and activism in Spain, even as infirmity and illness have been further underscored as a means of control over non-normative bodies and lives. This type of body politics has catalyzed Spanish queerness in a number of ways, as highlighted throughout this chapter, and reached its apotheosis in the 1990s in direct response to AIDS. Addressing the shifting social landscape of activism at this time, Llamas and Vila note that

> Ya en la década de los 90, el nuevo activismo lésbico y gay de grupos como LSD y La Radical Gai va a establecer una aproximación crítica a los mecanismos por los que un sistema de homofobia determina la vida y la muerte física o social de quienes encarnan la disidencia. Mientras la mayor parte del movimiento se vuelve hacia las abstracciones legales y los principios éticos, una corriente nueva vuelve a otorgar importancia a la presencia social, a la visibilidad, a la gestión de los placeres, a los intercambios corporales. El conocimiento, la autodeterminación y la difusión del cuerpo como sede de nuestros sexos-géneros, como geografía se ubican y se manifiestan el placer y el dolor, adquieren una importancia decisiva en las luchas de lesbianas y gays. La dimensión carnal de las vidas de lesbianas y gays pasa a ser un espacio de resistencia y de subversión. 'Lo personal es político' se expande con 'lo corporal es político'. (1994, 215)[17]

17 'By the 1990s, the new lesbian and gay activism of groups such as LSD and La Radical Gai begins to establish a critical approach to the mechanisms by which a homophobic system determines the life and physical or social death of those who embody dissent. While most of the movement turns to legal abstractions and ethical principles, a new trend once again gives importance to social presence, visibility, the management of pleasure, and bodily exchanges. Knowledge, self-determination, and the diffusion of the body as the seat of our sexes/genders and as a geography where pleasure and pain are located and are manifested, all acquire a decisive importance in the struggles of lesbians and gays. The embodied dimension of the lives of lesbians and gays becomes a space of resistance and subversion. "The personal is political" expands to "the corporeal is political".'

This brief detour into the 'future', as it were, and past the earliest years of AIDS in Spain shows the increasing influence of corporeal politics in the composition of queer activism. Llamas and Vila's compelling analysis underscores the growing importance of the body in the evolution of LGBTQ activism in Spain—not only in the pleasurable exchange between bodies but in the weaponized virulence of bodies in contact, and not only in the visibility of the political body but in the absence of those who have died and the pain of bodies breaking down in illness.

Ephemeral matters

Though the tactics and actions taken up by queer activist groups in the 1980s and 1990s as a means of visibilizing the queer body ('kiss-ins', 'die-ins', protests, or flyer distributions, among many others) strategically borrowed from the global tactics of resistance of groups like ACT UP or the Gay Men's Health Crisis, they were not new to Spain or Spanish queer resistance, as evidenced by a description of the 1934 procession of Las Carolinas given by de Fluvià (and briefly referenced earlier in this chapter). The strategies, methods, and actions of queer groups in Spain thus have localized histories of active political resistance as well as global ties to nascent and ongoing queer movements across the globe. This is made most evident in the AIDS-related ephemera and texts of groups like EHGAM (Euskal Heriak Gay Askapen Mugimendua) and various anti-AIDS organizations across Spain, as well as in noted artists like Nazario, all of whom help to make apparent just how visual culture and its ephemera have been utilized as a means to corporealize their sexualities. Such responses were varied, both in their earliest occurrences and in the latter years of the decade. Turning to a scattered collection of archival ephemera from the 1980s, then, illustrates the movements of queer organizations working against state control and containment, as well as the ways in which they responded to further containment on the basis of so-called medical fact.

By examining the earliest examples of this small archive of queer ephemera—a poster for the 1982 celebrations of gay pride in Spain, a program of the events and lectures that took place during Bilbao's pride demonstration that same year, and a manifesto circulated by EHGAM in 1985 in Bilbao—it becomes apparent just how images of the queer body were taken up in defense of visibility and freedom from oppression. On a poster for the 1982 celebration of a 'Día internacional del orgullo gai', for example, the title proudly proclaims 'NI REPRESIÓN / NI DISCRIMINACIÓN / TAL COMO ERES GANA LA CALLE' (Coordinadora de Frentes de Liberación Homosexual del Estado Español 1982), a clear call for queer public visibility. Indeed, in the imperative to 'gana[r] la calle', the flyer urges its readers to win back or occupy the streets in a call for physical action and a refusal to allow the containment or control of one's body, even if only for one day. Underneath this text is a list of the seven organizing activist groups,[18] all of which were in turn member organizations of the Coordinadora de Frentes de Liberación Homosexual del Estado Español (COFLHEE). This paragraph of text is bordered with '27 JUNIO DIA INTERNACIONAL DEL ORGULLO GAI' in Spanish, Galician, Basque, and Catalan, which ties together local queer struggles in Spain's variant regions to a common goal of visibility in the face of discrimination. The top three-fourths of the poster, meanwhile, is occupied by a striking image that frames visibility and physicality in a more playful, sexual way: an image showing the lower bodies of two male soccer players in brightly contrasting pink and white. The figure in a bright pink shirt leans suggestively against the other in the middle of a play for a pink football; his muscular legs tangled up with the other's, he reaches his hand into his opponent's impressively short shorts, grabbing his crotch. His shorts, in turn, feature a suggestive bulge.

The program for the 1982 'Día de Orgullo Gay' in Bilbao—part of the same celebrations as the first poster—centers sexuality and physicality in very similar ways. Underneath the name of the organization and 'Gay Harrotasunaren Eguna 82 Ekaina' / 'Día de Orgullo Gay 82 junio' is EHGAM's logo, the spike of an inverted triangle pointing to a pair of hands that reach out to each other in apparent longing, fingertips nearly touching. These hands are an outline of those of Adam and God from Michelangelo's *The Creation of Adam* (1512). The interior of the program includes a talk on 'machismo y homosexualidad' by Empar Pineda, a poetry recital, a marathon of gay cinema, an excursion to the countryside, and a talk on 'homosexualidad y legalidad' by Juan Mari Bandrés (which, according to the program, was only to be held in the event of not receiving authorization for the planned demonstration). The back page of the program includes a single, small image in the center of the page: a drawing of two men kissing passionately, their eyes closed. Underneath their mouths, and in the space between their bodies, the words 'apur dezagun araua' are written in Basque: 'return to yourself', the image urges.

The playful sexuality in the images on the program and poster seems almost at odds with the overt political tone of their texts, and one might be

18 The listed groups are Coordinadora de Colectivos Gais de Galicia (CCGG), Euskal Herriak Gay Aspaken Mugimendua (EHGAM), Frente de Liberación Homosexual de Andalucía (FLHA), Frente de Liberación Homosexual de Castilla (FLHOC), Front d'Alliberament Gai de Catalunya (FAGC), Grupo de Acción para la Liberación Homosexual (GALHO), and Moviment d'Alliberament Gai del Pais Valencià (MAGPV).

tempted to see the footballers' bodies groping and crashing into each other as undermining the serious work of the events' demonstrations, events, and lectures. But as I hope to have shown throughout this chapter, sex and activism have long been closely linked, each responding to the limits imposed and oppositional forces enacted upon the other. The passionate kiss between the two men on the 1982 Bilbao gay pride program, in this way, implores its readers to 'return to [themselves]' by looping together visibility, sexual desire, and personhood into the same framework. Such a move is possible not the least through the suggestion that its queer interlocutors have been lost or waylaid by silence and sexual repression. Seen together, then, the beefy footballers and passionate kissers reframe queer visibility as sexual empowerment and activism and in direct response to the legal, medical, and discursive control over queer bodies, a control which had filtered through public discourse and institutional apparatuses in equal measure. Enacting one's sexuality through visibility and displaying it proudly (even brazenly, perhaps) was a way to empower oneself, the LGBTQ community, and queer activism in Spain.

As seen in earlier chapters, 1982 was in some ways too early for the most urgent work on AIDS to have made its way into queer media in Spain, much less popular discourse of any kind. This began to change in the years following and, as the urgency (and institutional silence) grew, the corporealization of queer politics took a new turn. On June 27, 1985, as part of the celebrations aoround the 'Día mundial de la liberación gay y lesbiana in Bilbao', EHGAM distributed a manifesto that traced a brief history of queer activist work in the Basque Country and set forth a list of demands and complaints to local and state authorities. The flyer is carefully typed out, with thick handwriting across the top of the sheet: '27 JUNIO / DIA MUNDIAL DE LA LIBERACION GAY Y LESBIANA / BILBAO 1985.' On the other side, the document has been translated into Basque. Decrying the homophobia and superficial tolerance of the Spanish government, the flyer argues that 'estamos en el reino de la tolerancia en donde los gais y las lesbianas pueden existir siempre y cuando no se sepa, no se diga o se mantengan lejos. El desprecio y la burla suelen acompañar a quien no esconde su homosexualidad' [we are in the kingdom of tolerance, in which gays and lesbians can exist as long as they go unnoticed, are not talked about, and stay far away. Disdain and mockery tend to follow those who do not hide their homosexuality] (EHGAM 1985). With this critique, EHGAM called attention to the purported tolerance proffered to LGBTQ individuals and communities as another means of social exclusion and control, one which pathologized queerness as the product of one's aberrant sex, sexuality, or gender. After listing further demands (the creation of an anti-discrimination law and the rejection of another law which could be used to expel queer individuals from the army), the group makes a final denunciation of 'la indiferencia de las autoridades sanitarias ante el alarmismo y el sensacionalismo anti-gay por motivo del SIDA, que tampoco se aborda con una política de prevención seria y responsible' [the indifference of health authorities to alarmism and anti-gay sensationalism due to AIDS, which is also not addressed with a serious and responsible prevention policy] (EHGAM 1985). At the bottom of the document is EHGAM's logo: an inverted triangle with a lower-case lambda in its center. The name of the group borders the triangle's top line. Alongside the logo is a bulleted series of demands that both summarize the flyer and suggest even larger struggles. These are, among others, 'CONTRA EL MACHISMO / DERECHO AL PROPIO CUERPO... / DERECHO A UNA INFORMACIÓN NO MACHISTA NI PATRIARCAL EN LOS MEDIOS DE LA COMUNICACIÓN' [AGAINST MACHISMO / THE RIGHT TO ONE'S OWN BODY... / THE RIGHT TO NON-MACHO OR PATRIARCHAL INFORMATION IN THE MEDIA] (EHGAM 1985).

EHGAM's flyer clearly indicates its place in a global struggle for queer rights and lives while powerfully situating its fight against localized discriminatory practices and culturally specific institutional biases. By drawing on global symbols of queerness, it connects up to histories of discrimination and activism in solidarity; that is, its celebration of a 'gay liberation day' (also known as Christopher Street Day and, eventually, [Gay] Pride) takes up the legacy of the 1969 Stonewall riots in New York City; the inverted triangle in its logo references the mass murder and extermination of homosexuals in the Holocaust; and the lower-case lambda is a symbol of queer activism put into use by gay activist groups in New York City in the early 1970s. The text of the flyer makes similar claims to localized struggles and their more global counterparts, both in the proposal of an anti-discriminatory law modeled on French laws of the time and in reference to the ongoing AIDS epidemic. Interestingly, such a globalizing move is in lockstep with some of the discriminatory practices that calcified the image of HIV/AIDS as a 'gay plague' in Spain; that is, by linking up to queer activist practices across the globe and drawing on a sort of shared symbology of queerness, groups like EHGAM perhaps unwittingly reinforced epidemiological similarities across communities. Thus, and even as they no doubt found the fight for queer liberation invigorated by cross-cultural synergies, they reified the global similarities of HIV/AIDS, despite the fact that it was emphatically not the same in Spain as it was in the United States—neither in its timeline, affected groups, nor epidemiological spread.

That said, there is no doubt that the alternative would have been worse—by decoupling their fight from other groups and communities across the globe, these Spanish organizations would have been embracing instead silence and death, to paraphrase the evergreen ACT UP slogan. For that reason, perhaps, much queer activist ephemera that emerged from the latter half of this period in Spain (from 1985 to the early 1990s, roughly) turns to similar campaigns of awareness, treatment, and prevention as those found in other communities across the globe. These campaigns, in turn, broadened their focus to include women, encouraged safe sex by promoting condom usage, and promoted clean needle exchanges. Such strategies were wholly compatible with the corporealization of queer activism in Spain, not only in their clear attempts to promote the diversity of experiences and to limit attempts at containment, but also in their ethical origins; in other words, the concern for the body as site of transgressive promise was nothing new to the LGBTQ community in Spain, and campaigns and strategies that highlighted the inherent pleasures and pains of sexual intimacy and contact with others only furthered the visibility of queer bodies. For these reasons, the move to examine AIDS through such strategic foci in the late 1980s and early 1990s may have seemed a sensible—if not necessarily radical—way to make queer sex and queer bodies visible while also producing a tactical jab that limited the spread of AIDS's infectious reach.

All of this is most clearly seen in the fact that even avowed anarchists and 'radicals' of the queer punk scene of the Spanish *Movida* took up the call for safer sex, clean needles, and healthier living. This seems somewhat counterintuitive to what we know of the late *Movida*, the legacy of which has often been overpopulated with tales of hedonistic nightlife and drug use. Nevertheless, the move to safe sex campaigning demonstrates just how virulent the spread of the illness had become among the clusters of queer artists and drug users in youth culture at the time. Nazario, for example, whose famed queer comics were nearly ubiquitous in the 1980s, offered his talent to safe sex campaigns like that of 'Folla seguro, o el Misterio de Navón', part of a late 1980s campaign by the group Gais per la Salut (GPS). Nazario's comic consists of two pages of five loosely connected vignettes, each of which demonstrates a variety of reactions to safe sex campaigns of the time. The panels show groups of anthropomorphic penises discussing medical rumor and fact, practicing or advocating for safe sex, and arguing over what 'good sex' can look like. As would be the case with other promotional campaigns of the time, 'Folla seguro' expends a deal of educational energy convincing its readers that safe sex can, in fact, be good, fun, and sexy. It also shows its main characters refusing condomless sex as well as the ingestion of any bodily fluids, offering up tactics for abstaining from the theoretically unsafe practices[19] that would increase their chance of transmission of HIV.

In the first panel, two penises are shown lounging in the private space of a home. One of the two leans casually against a wall, smoking a cigarette. He wears a long, open coat, revealing his shaft-torso and the bumpy scrotum from which his crossed legs emerge. A scarf is tightly tied around his neck, which is situated just beneath his glans, and a short, trimmed moustache covers his frenulum/face; in a hand that is cocked on his 'hip' he holds a small bag. His uncircumcised companion is stretched out on a chair, covered in a patterned robe and smoking a pipe. He wears glasses as he reads the newspaper. The standing character asks his friend, '¿Entonces, no es verdad que el SIDA se contagia con la saliva, besándose, o haciendo pajas o chupando pollas o bebiendo en el mismo vaso?' [So, it's not true that AIDS is spread by saliva, kissing, or jerking off or sucking cocks or drinking from the same glass?] Without looking up from his paper, the lounging penis replies: '¡Todo eso son falsedades y alarmismos! La enfermedad solo se transmite si hay contacto entre sangre y sangre como en el caso de usar la misma jeringuilla, máquina de afeitar, o cepillo de dientes; o si hay contacto directo entre el semen y la sangre' [All of these are falsehoods and scaremongering! The disease is only transmitted if there is contact between blood and blood, as in the case of using the same syringe, razor, or toothbrush; or if there is direct contact between semen and blood] (Nazario 1987). This conversation, which woodenly reads as if it were lifted from a medical pamphlet, reveals the clear didactic intentions of Nazario and Gais per la Salut; even so, the sexual playfulness of the image is telegraphed through its queerly coded characters and tongue-in-cheek imagery. Like the humor of Las Pekinesas and 'SIDA da', the effect of seeing an uncut penis dressed in a foreskin turtleneck and luxuriously stretched out on a flowered chair is at once playful and educational, meaningful and ludicrous.

Underneath this short vignette is a longer panel of a scene in a gay bar. Six characters are shown engaged in separate conversations: a leather daddy and a friend in bondage gear, two queens chatting, a short, solitary loner, and a bartender in folkloric drag. All of these characters have little moustaches,

19 I say 'theoretically' unsafe only because some of the information on HIV/AIDS that is presented as medical fact is not entirely correct, as was quite typical of the 1980s. Even as physicians were still learning about the syndrome, public information campaigns often relied on early guesswork, which sometimes produced a sort of telephone game of partial truth. Nazario's comic dabbles in this by decrying oral sex without a condom as highly unsafe and by presenting competing medical claims to the validity of the antibody test. In this case, the former is untrue, and the latter is only partially so.

a nod to gay male fashions of the time as well as a clear indicator of their gender, and all of them are wearing sunglasses, which might be a way to avoid the peculiar problem of figuring out where a set of eyes might actually be located on an anthropomorphized penis. Some of the characters smoke, others have drinks in front of them, and some wear accessories like belts, pearl necklaces, leather jackets, or leather boots. Littered on the floor of the bar are used condoms. From left to right, the conversation between the leather daddy and his buddy in bondage gear appears first. Following conventional medical wisdom of the time, the daddy notes: 'Dicen que usar la misma maquinilla de afeitar puede ser tan peligroso como usar la misma jeringuilla. Lo de usar el mismo cepillo me parece una guarrería' [They say that using the same razor can be just as dangerous as using the same syringe. Using the same brush seems like a disgusting mess to me.] The character in bondage playfully propositions him in return: '¿Nos vamos un ratito a mi casa a usar la misma cama? ¡Tengo unos condones fantásticos!' [Shall we go to my house for a little while to use the same bed? I have some great condoms!] The two queens at the other end of the bar, meanwhile, squeal at each other as one remarks on the smoothness of his skin:

> ¡Mira qué cutis! ¡Toca! ¿Sabes qué crema uso? ¡Mmmh! La llamo 'Misterio' de la Casa 'Navón'. Verás, cuando se la chupo a alguien, en lugar de tragarme la leche (que puede ser peligroso) procuro que se me corran en la cara. ¡Mira, ni una arruga![20]

His friend finds this all-natural method tremendously appealing, and definitely preferable to his previously preferred method of spitting out his partners' semen.

Further panels show a number of scenes that advocate condom usage: a character who initially refuses to put on a condom because he is clearly 'una polla muy sana' [a very healthy cock], and his partner, who convinces him that health is not an inherent trait but a practice; another character faces a line of glory holes from which condom-covered penises emerge and, seeing a bare penis, chastises it angrily for not wearing its 'raincoat'; a couple who have been together for 35 years, who lovingly promise their fidelity to one another but still promise to use a condom if they were to ever sleep with anyone else; and finally, the only human figure, naked except for a boa and a condom on his sizeable member. This last character is wreathed by a

20 'Look at this complexion! Touch it! Do you know what cream I use? Mmmh! I call it "Mystery" of the House "Navón". You see, when I suck someone off, instead of swallowing their load (which can be dangerous) I get them to cum on my face. Look, not one wrinkle!'

halo, one arm on his hip and the other pointing to the sky as he proclaims '¡Follemos y al cielo iremos, pero seguro!' [Let's fuck and we'll go to heaven for sure!] Underneath is a prayer to this carnal saint: 'San Pollardino de la Gloriosa Metida, líbranos a todas de la sífilis y el SIDA' [Saint Priapus of the Heavenly Lay, deliver us all from syphilis and AIDS] (Nazario 1987).

There is much to say about the very queer pleasures and sexual escapades seen in 'Folla seguro', but most important is the recurrence to these characters' fleshly desires and their attempts to have good, fun sex. In this way, the comic's subtitle, 'El misterio de Navón', teasingly alludes to the comic's primary premise; that is, 'Navón' is both a light play on Avon cosmetics and a suggestive reference to Spanish slang for a large penis, and its 'mystery' is the 'cream' that it produces. Although it is, perhaps, designed to be little more than a throwaway joke nestled in one of the comic's panels, the linkage of semen to 'mystery' further underscores some of the deep-seated anxieties surrounding sex that the comic works hard to soothe. That is, these mortal fears about what one's semen can do to another person become knotted with tension, wrapped up as they are with queer sexual pleasures and practices that had previously been liberational; medical recommendations, on the other hand, were either unclear, uninformed, or unheard of, and they produced a cascading sense of confusion among friends and groups, who were often forced to take charge of their own sexual health and education. 'El misterio de Navón' serves as a clear attempt to demystify safe sex in the late 1980s and early 1990s by making it seem just as fun, raunchy, and sex positive as queer sex practices prior to the onslaught of the epidemic. At the same time, however, it inadvertently equates sex with mystery, uneasily addressing the range of popular beliefs around HIV/AIDS and sex.

As evidenced by Nazario's comic, the call to safe (or safer) sex was increasingly taken up at this time, partly in response to the corporealization of queer activism and politics, and partly because queer men just weren't as accustomed to using condoms. As Óscar Guasch notes, 'con anterioridad a 1985 el número de homosexuales españoles que practican el sexo seguro era escaso; en adelante esa cifra aumentará' [Before 1985, the number of Spanish homosexuals who practiced safe sex was low; henceforth that figure would increase] (1991, 81). He does footnote this comment somewhat ruefully: 'decir que los homosexuales españoles practican "sexo seguro" es sin duda excesivo, porque lo que se entiende por tal engloba muchas más precauciones que las que ejecuta el homosexual de nuestro país' [To say that Spanish homosexuals practice 'safe sex' is undoubtedly an exaggeration, because what is understood as such includes far more precautions than those carried out by the homosexual in our country] (1991, 81). By this, Guasch is in part focusing on condom usage and anal sex, which he states was quite commonly understood and to a large extent utilized by the early 1990s, although its ubiquity did produce some uncertainty around other types of sex (analingus, cunnilingus, and fellatio, for example) and their potential to transmit HIV. He writes that

> el *sexo seguro* define algo mucho más amplio que el empleo del preservativo en el coito. Sobre este tema, sobre sexo seguro, la información que manejan los homosexuales españoles es muy deficiente, y ello incide en su praxis sexual cotidiana del siguiente modo: primero, la felación sin preservativo sigue practicándose de forma indiscriminada (si bien se evita la eyaculación en la boca); segundo, la realización o no del beso anal, tiene que ver más con el asco que pueda producir que con el conocimiento de que es una práctica de riesgo; y, tercero, una práctica sexual común es la de realizar el coito anal sin preservativo evitando eyacular en el compañero, o bien colocar el preservativo para permitir lo anterior tras una penetración previa sin él. (Guasch 1991, 82)[21]

Much of what Guasch notes here is a failure to plainly and explicitly communicate what safe sex meant, which many larger and more official campaigns balked at, as we will see. Nazario's 'El misterio de Navón' is interesting in this aspect, as it attempts to speak directly to its targeted audience via explicit imagery, commonly used queer slang, and up-to-date medical information.

Nazario's work was not alone, as a number of activist groups and regional anti-AIDS committees created flyers and distributed information that addressed the queer community directly and openly. In an undated flyer from the Asociación Ciudadana Anti-SIDA de Málaga (ASIMA), the topic of what safe sex means for women and lesbians is openly addressed, delineating safe versus unsafe sex as well as what pleasure in an epidemic can look like.[22] On the flyer, a handwritten title, 'Lesbianas y SIDA', is placed

21 'Safe sex defines something much broader than the use of a condom during intercourse. On this topic—safe sex—the information that Spanish homosexuals have is very lacking, and this affects their daily sexual practice in the following way: first, fellatio without a condom continues to be practiced indiscriminately (although oral ejaculation is avoided); second, whether or not rimming is performed has more to do with the disgust it may produce than with the knowledge that it is a risky practice; and, third, a common sexual practice is to perform anal intercourse without a condom, avoiding ejaculation on the partner, or to place the condom to allow the above after having anal sex without it.'

22 Though it is undated, the medical information and knowledge available—in addition to its references to HIV, which was only named as such in 1986—suggest that this flyer was distributed in the early 1990s.

next to a photocopied image of a bare-breasted woman's torso. Inside the tri-fold flyer is a description of AIDS and HIV and a brief acknowledgment of medical misinformation: 'La forma de contagio ha sido fuente de especulaciones alarmista [*sic*] y tendenciosas' [The form of contagion has been a source of alarmist and biased speculations] (Asociación Ciudadana Anti-SIDA de Málaga, n.d.). It continues by noting what is certain, which are specific practices known to transmit HIV—among these, needle sharing, transfusions, mother-to-child transmission during birth and breastfeeding, and unsafe sex. Centering female sexuality, the flyer discusses unsafe sex practices of particular relevance to women, safe sex acts, and multiple partners of varying genders.

A fluorescent pink flyer from Gais per la Salut released in summer of 1987 seeks an even wider audience by including its information in six different languages (Catalan, Spanish, Italian, English, German, and French). This small flyer is about the size of a note card and is folded six times, with a single paragraph of information that is repeated in a different language on each side. Under a campaign titled 'Estima com vulguis / Estima Segur' [Love as you want / Love Safely], the group writes that

> el verano y las vacaciones son el tiempo de los viajes, de nuevos contactos y amistades. Seguramente ya habrás oído hablar del problema del SIDA y de que esta enfermedad tiene más incidentes en unos países como en otros, como también unos gobiernos han realizado mejores campanas de prevención que otros. En Catalunya tenemos mucho que aprender de otros países respecto a la información para prevenir el SIDA, y por esto, ante la poca iniciativa de la Administración se ha formado Gais per la Salut. (Gais per la Salut 1987)[23]

Playing to an audience of summer tourists to Spain (and to a burgeoning industry of queer tourism), the campaign highlights the local and the global by underscoring the unequal treatment of HIV/AIDS across countries and critiquing the inaction of the local government of Cataluña itself. Tying these concerns together by euphemistically acknowledging the fact of sex itself, the new contacts and friendships that result from a tourist's hot summer

23 'Summer and holidays are the time of travel, of new contacts and friendships. Surely you have already heard about the problem of AIDS and that this disease has more incidents in some countries than in others, as well as the fact that some governments have carried out better prevention campaigns than others. In Catalonia we have a lot to learn from other countries regarding information to prevent AIDS, and for this reason, given the scarce initiative of the Administration, Gais per la Salut was formed.'

nights in Spain, Gais per la Salut sees HIV/AIDS as intimately connected to queer sexual lives and queer sex.

They are, however, understandably resistant to the institutional language of the time that demarcates the LGBTQ community as a particular 'risk group', a technique discussed at length in this chapter and throughout this book. They write: 'Obviamente el SIDA es una enfermedad que se transmite por una serie de prácticas de riesgo, y rechazamos la acusación discriminatoria de ser llamados "grupos de riesgo" como culpables, como hacen Reagan, el Gobierno de Baviera, Le Pen en Francia y todos los reaccionarios del mundo' [Obviously AIDS is a disease that is transmitted by a series of risky practices, and we reject the discriminatory accusation of being called 'risk groups' as if we are guilty, as Reagan, the government of Bavaria, Le Pen in France and all the reactionaries of the world do] (Gais per la Salut 1987). This motley crew of 'reactionaries of the world' highlights some of the more notorious examples of institutional and legal discrimination during this time by drawing attention to governments and their use of language to corral queers into certain limited spaces. The flyer also delineates safe practices from risky, touting the condom as a universal equalizer. Ultimately, in a pandemic that was both local and global, and with noted bad actors who recur to institutional and longstanding modes of discrimination, one of the ways that GPS resists is by shifting the focus from people to practices and offering safe(r) ways of connection. As a way to underscore this idea, the flyer places a small hand-drawn national or local icon next to each paragraph. These icons—a range of symbols or statues that are iconic to each country or place—are each shown covered by a giant condom. The symbols are, in order of appearance: the Columbus Monument (Barcelona), the Statue of the Bear and the Strawberry Tree (Madrid), the Tower of Pisa (Italy), Big Ben (England), the Brandenburg Gate (Germany), and the Eiffel Tower (France). With few exceptions, most of these buildings are immediately recognizable (and recognizably phallic) symbols of countries and cities. Covering these symbols in condoms is an admittedly simplistic—but impactful—way to link queer communities across countries and to move toward minimizing risky practices which could lead to the spread of HIV/AIDS. In the absence of clear safe sex campaigns from any number of state institutions—in fact, given the clear anti-queer rhetoric from many of these countries—the GPS flyer advocates for sexuality at the same time that it recognizes risk and viral transmission.

Sí da, No da

The cluster and range of queer-produced ephemera analyzed above showcases reactions from the LGBTQ communities to a history of systematic oppression and the ongoing placement of queer communities in harm's way. By examining this ephemera, early news reports, and activist responses, it becomes increasingly clear that queer communities and activist groups were forced to create safe sex and anti-AIDS campaigns on their own, while facing overwhelming governmental and institutional inaction. Such inaction might seem at odds with the assertion of constant vigilance and policing by state authorities, but silence—like humor—can be a method of control over subcultures and minority groups. It is clear that the lack of centralized governmental response certainly accelerated the spread of HIV/AIDS. Still, campaigns like the ones carried out by the queer activist groups above had positive outcomes that an official and more generalized campaign could not have had. This is to say that these queer-produced ephemera were able to reach a broad group of people where they were, be it in bars, sex clubs, monthly meetings, or on the streets, while also performing a handful of vital community functions: they provided clear medical information, combating the silence and misinformation circulating among communities; they educated queer folks on the definition and practice of safe sex; and they worked to center queer sexualities as good, pleasurable, and not inherently risky.

Governmental campaigns were rarely this refined, in part due to their long history of coupling queerness and risk, and in part perhaps because they saw themselves as beholden to a wider audience that saw itself as distinct from (and mostly oppositional to) the so-called risk groups of HIV/AIDS. As Keller and Snyder note,

> public health announcements from Spain's Ministerio de Sanidad y Consumo only began promoting condom usage exclusively as a measure to prevent HIV transmission in 1994, whereas previous campaigns arguably participated in the social marginalization of at-risk groups by labelling AIDS synonymous with homosexuality and intravenous drug use. (2011, 94)

Perhaps the best-known governmental effort in these early years was the 'Sí da / No da' campaign, which was released in 1989 across a variety of media, including posters and television spots. Divided into risky actions that cause ('sí da') versus those that do not cause ('no da') AIDS, the campaign playfully depicts a series of anthropomorphized male and female symbols performing a wide variety of daily actions; of these, sharing shaving razors, needles, and toothbrushes, mother-child interactions, unsterile tattoos, and sex with carriers are all touted as risky actions that 'give' AIDS. In contrast, actions that can't cause/give AIDS are using condoms, swimming with, playing with, or using the same bathrooms as carriers, insect bites, drinking from the same glass, shaking hands, kissing or hugging, and wearing someone else's clothes. The seropositive symbols wear the words SIDA emblazoned on their chests, an image that Keller and Snyder critique thoroughly:

> By labelling the figures with 'SIDA' the poster conflates 'disease' with cartoonish representations of practices that are visually collapsed into 'junkies' and 'homosexuals' (i.e., from 'gay sex "sí, da [SIDA]"'; to 'gays are AIDS carriers'), further undermining a sense of public awareness that might encourage collective responsibility in preventing HIV transmission. (2011, 95)

The campaign has been further critiqued by Alberto Mira, who writes that 'so humorous and underplayed was this campaign ... that its effect was negligible' (qtd. in Smith 1996, 107).

This campaign, the first in a string of campaigns in Spain,[24] shares similarities with several of the queer ephemera seen throughout this chapter: it brings humor to bear on a decidedly unfunny epidemic, it anthropomorphizes select figures in sexualized situations, and it toys with linguistic expression and wordplay. Though much of this might be circumstantial, the control over language from a place of institutional power is far from casual. Over the course of this chapter, I have attempted to underscore the long history of definitional practices over queerness—the story of who is afforded control over meaning, and what such control means for those who are being named. The ability to define an experience, group of people, or even a pandemic means that naming practices adhere to dominant paradigms of power. This is how the term 'GRID' came into being, the reason why 'gay cancer' was so frequently used in these early years, and how queerness, crime, and illness are so linked throughout the history of Spain.

Understanding the history of state responses to queerness—and the ways that institutions controlled the public meaning and response to the LGBTQ community—shows that even a well-intentioned and helpful campaign such as 'Sí da' could be part of a system that distorts queerness. To be clear, there is nothing particularly insidious about the 'Sí da' campaign. That is,

24 This includes the famous 'Póntelo, Pónselo' [Put it on yourself, Put it on him] campaigns, among others. Belén Remacha (2019) provides a short overview of similarly impactful AIDS campaigns in Spain in recent decades.

it toys with language, playfully using an easy linguistic device alongside bright, simple drawings in a way that would be easily memorable for a wide audience; it attempts to control the narrative of AIDS, harnessing language in a way that can serve an educational purpose; it is informative, meaningful, and likely had some sort of impact on its audience. Still, I think of the performance of Las Pekinesas, which is almost none of these things. 'SIDA da' is unruly and chaotic, it is invested with both nonsense and heavy, coded meanings, and it is distinctly queer in its mode of delivery and references. It resists the confines of language, and attempts to articulate a half-thought, something that is only emerging, something that may not be articulable. The performance of Las Pekinesas plays to the humor of a community at risk from within that community itself, critiquing institutions and supporting queerness. The government's 'Sí da' campaign promotes action and education, stripping away the raw messiness of sexuality, queer or not. It is sanitized, fit for mass consumption. For these reasons, the history of reading queerness as hypersexualized and predatorial serves as a backdrop for the 'Sí da' campaign, which can only articulate itself in opposition to queer infirmity.

'Si da', then, stands in stark contrast to the ways that queerness has articulated its struggles against a range of dominant institutions. That is, from the work of de Fluvià against dictatorial anti-homosexuality laws to the anti-AIDS groups and activism of the early 1980s, the queer ephemera that we have seen over the length of this chapter is unambiguously sexualized: queer bodies are laid bare, they come into close contact, and they sensuously connect. We see such sexuality in Nazario's talking penises, the bare-breasted woman of the 'Lesbianas y SIDA' flyer, and in the EHGAM flyers, all of which openly foreground sexuality, its desirability, and pleasurable ways of continuing to have sex in an epidemic. These ephemera rage against normalization and the constant policing of queerness by the state and its institutions, underscoring the ways in which the messy physicality of sex resists utility. Though the emphasis on the exaggerated sexuality of queer folks aligns with the state's naming and policing practices, the unfettered recurrence to pleasure in pandemic times sets these ephemera apart. This is in line with Ricardo Llamas, who claims that 'si bien la realidad humana es (de manera general e indiscutiblemente) corpórea, podría decirse que "algunas personas son más cuerpo que otras"' [Although human reality is (in a general and indisputable way) corporeal, it could be said that 'some people are more of a body than others'] (1994, 142). Possessing 'more body' than others is another way of drawing attention to the physicality of queerness, its proximity to health and illness, and how sex is always tied up into all of these.

Llamas also insists that 'es desde el cuerpo desde donde debe lucharse, tanto contra los criterios de reducción discriminatoria y dominación como contra la mismísima pandemia' [it is from the body where one must fight, both against the criteria of discriminatory reduction and domination as well as against the pandemic itself] (1994, 142). Fighting from this place of sick embodiment harnesses what's queer about feeling sick, from those sexual practices by which queer folks have long been vilified, made infirm, and punished. The laws that normalize sexuality must, by their very nature, name and define abnormality. By recentering the body and queer sexuality, AIDS activism attempted to take control of these definitional practices, coming up with new ways of articulating the pleasures and risks of sex. Sometimes these images borrow from the language and structures of the time, as in the case of much of the EHGAM materials, and sometimes they repurpose medical information in queer formats, as with the comic by Nazario and GPS; other times the words spin out and into the air, queerly toyed with in ways both painful and pleasurable. This moment of articulation—of all of this, when queer folks in Spain were learning ways to take back the narratives of infirmity laid upon them—was crucial for the developing LGBTQ movement in Spain, for AIDS activism, and for the ways they understood sex.

CHAPTER FOUR

Into the Ruins

On June 25, 1985, under the headline 'Vecinos de Embajadores expulsan a unos delincuentes de un refugio ruinoso' [Neighbors of Embajadores expel criminals from a dilapidated shelter], journalist Esther Sánchez wrote about the efforts of a group of neighbors in Madrid to forcibly evict squatters from their neighborhood and, more concretely, from the ruins of an old convent. Denouncing the inaction of the police, who had turned a blind eye to the neighborhood violence despite frequent and deadly attacks, Sánchez frames the efforts of the neighbors as heroic while maligning the squatters, writing: 'En estas ruinas han encontrado refugio todo tipo de vagabundos y delincuentes, que entre tabiques semiderruidos y al abrigo del agua y del sol han instalado colchones y mantas para protegerse incluso de las "miradas indiscretas"' [In these ruins all kinds of homeless people and criminals have found refuge, who between semi-ruined partitions and sheltered from water and sun have installed mattresses and blankets to protect themselves even from 'prying eyes'] (1985, 43). Free from such outside prying eyes, the squatters 'tienen atemorizado al barrio: amenazas, robos, navajazos ... están a la orden del día' [they have terrorized the neighborhood: threats, robberies, knives ... are the order of the day], Sánchez reports (1985, 43). She continues by noting that, after the stabbing of a local bar owner and a robbery at a bakery, 'un grupo de vecinos se dirigieron de forma pacífica a las ruinas y quemaron todas las mantas, colchones, jeringuillas' [a group of neighbors went peacefully to the ruins and burned all the blankets, mattresses, syringes] (1985, 43).

The article tells a story of a neighborhood under siege. Its framing clearly sets the neighborhood 'locals' up against the homeless outsiders, who are positioned as emphatically not part of the neighborhood themselves. What's more, Sánchez writes that the neighbors 'se consideran un grupo de amigos que se hacen fuertes agrupándose contra estos intrusos que amenazan la seguridad barrio' [consider themselves a group of friends who become strong by grouping together against these intruders who threaten neighborhood security] (1985, 43). Envisioning the vigilante collective of neighbors as a group of 'friends' up against dangerous packs of 'intruders' paints homelessness and drug use as producing decidedly criminal behaviors that must be quelled, even when local authorities will not or cannot intervene satisfactorily. This is not to ignore the actual crimes being committed in the neighborhood or to dismiss the groups' fears outright, but it is important to understand how these things—drug use, homelessness, and crime writ large—become framed as decidedly non-native to this space.

This type of vandalism and street violence was fairly common in the Madrid of the Transition, with the areas comprising Embajadores and La Latina receiving a great deal of notoriety during this period. In the Sánchez article, the president of the local Business Owners' Association points to a specific space as the origin of the troubles in Embajadores, angrily grumbling that 'todo esto tiene su foco en las ruinas del convento, que según nuestro alcalde son un tesoro y, por eso, no se tiran. Ayer pusieron unas vallas, pero no sabemos si servirá para algo' [the source of all of this is the ruins of the convent, which according to our mayor are a treasure and so they're not brought down. Yesterday they put up some fences, but we don't know if it will serve any purpose] (Sánchez 1985, 43). Seeing the site as both potentially emblematic of the neighborhood (the historical treasure that the ruins represent) and exceptional to it (separated by a fence, a ruined eyesore), the area is configured as neither here nor there, part of the neighborhood and a locus of otherness.

The ruins in question were part of the Escuelas Pías de San Fernando, a space with a long and storied history in Madrid's religious and social life—though one might not have known much about its origins in the 1980s, or even today. The original complex was nearly the size of a city block, and consisted of a square, a convent, a school, and a few other buildings. Today, parts of the ruins have been conserved, another part serves as a playground and open-air market, and a large section has been converted to offices and a spacious library for the Universidad Nacional de Educación a Distancia. Remnants of the past still cling to the space, which has been renovated such as to preserve aspects of its former life: the nave of the church is visible and lined with books and pew-like carrels for study, there are cracked and crumbling pillars, and an arch leading to a circular rotunda, brightly lit and filled with plants and bookshelves. Underneath the modern fixtures and updates, the former ruins of the church are at once highlighted and transfigured. Whispers of its past frame the structure now as they did in the 1980s.

With its history of crime, vandalism, and transition, the ruined site of the Escuelas Pías in the 1980s is emblematic of the spaces to which people living with AIDS were relegated, as well as the role that space in general plays in history. By thinking through the spatial politics of AIDS in the 1980s, this chapter looks at how drug use was confined, treated, and represented at the time. In particular, I examine the spatial links between prisons and drug dens in order to think through the connections between AIDS, crime, and drugs. As in Chapters 2 and 3, the tropes of illegality, law breaking, and monstrosity were key components in representing AIDS in the early years of the epidemic. In this case, however, these components had powerful repercussions for the treatment and response to HIV/AIDS in Spain. That is to say that in Spain, unlike other countries, HIV/AIDS infection rates and new cases were often tied to drug use. For example, by September 30, 1985, drug users

> represented 8% of all European cases and were reported by nine countries ... Italy and Spain together accounted for 63% of the IV drug abusers with AIDS in Europe. Forty-five (49%) of the 92 Italian patients and 23 (37%) of the 63 Spanish patients were members of this risk group. (Centers for Disease Control and Prevention 1986)

In contrast, male homosexuals accounted for less than half of all known cases in Spain (hemophiliacs and drug users no doubt made up the larger percentage). Despite the public perception of AIDS as a 'gay disease' in the United States and Europe, the reality is that drug use was a major component in the story of HIV in Spain, even as drug users were made invisible in its narratives and ignored as they collapsed at one's feet.

News media and institutional campaigns, however, rarely underscored drug use or treatment as a key component in combating misunderstandings and misinformation about AIDS. Just as importantly, the outbreak narrative that developed around the illness very rarely saw drug users as anything but deadbeats who refused treatment and help and who were essentially lost causes. Documenting this process, this chapter examines several news reports on drug users and prisoners, noting how the portrayal of different risk groups holds to a well-established dichotomy between those who deserved illness (homosexuals and intravenous drug users) and those who didn't (hemophiliacs, children, the public at large). I frame this issue as one that is bound up with questions of space. That to say that there are spaces which people with AIDS were made to occupy and to which they were seen to belong—ruins. This chapter examines two specific examples of criminal 'ruins' that have been inflected by HIV/AIDS: the Escuelas Pías, which served as site of criminal activity in the 1980s and has since been rehabilitated, and Carabanchel Prison, a carceral space on the brink of collapse throughout the 1980s and which is now little more than debris. Frequently paired with HIV/AIDS, the 'ruin' became metaphorized in popular media of the time as indicative of the seropositive community at large, just another example of the ruinous and ruined lives that they were portrayed as living.

To think through these collapsing ruins and spaces in crisis, I follow Tim Edensor's work on memories and ruins, which analyzes 'how the effects of the disordered spaces of industrial ruins can interrogate and contest the normative ways in which memory is spatialized in the city' (2005, 829). I adapt Edensor's work to the Spanish spatial context, in which ruins have not historically been a product of industrial work but instead are the crumbling remnants of the ancient past (medieval churches, historic city centers, and more). I also draw upon the growing work done in Hispanic urban studies to consider the specificities of how these places were represented and configured in Spain. At its core, this chapter tells some of the narratives surrounding intravenous drug users, piecing the fragmented stories together to better understand the narrative constructed around HIV/AIDS risk groups in Spain.

The place of space

Returning to such seemingly disparate sites of AIDS in the 1980s is a complicated task, given that they have unique meanings and histories attached to them. This is to point out the obvious, perhaps, by noting that the drug den and the prison are utilized to different ends, are inhabited or abandoned for different reasons, and are used to mean different things socially. They are also not all ruins, though I will argue here that they circulate around a sort of politics of the ruin. That is, and as I explore later in this chapter, there existed a popular perception of ruins as connected to disorder—both as organizational lack and cancerous social illness. The neglect that ran rampant in prisons at the time in Spain (despite the promise of structured order offered within their walls) meant that both spaces circulated around states of disorder. These two types of spaces were also inhabited by intravenous drug users who passed through briefly in transit or who were made to stay for years, imprisoned. This connection is important, and it means that as the number of cases of HIV and AIDS rose in Spain, sites like these became increasingly associated with illness, disorder, and ruin.

In some of his work, Tim Edensor frames the search for meaning in ruins as an 'urge to seek out the ghosts of places', which is 'bound up with the politics of remembering the past and, more specifically, with the spatialisation of memory and how memory is sought, articulated, and inscribed upon space' (2005, 829). Though I find the ghostly analogies compelling, I am more concerned with histories of use, and how certain spaces become analogous to any number of surprising things—how a former convent like the Escuelas Pías becomes a symbol for AIDS, for example, a place to point to as a metaphorical ground zero of a virus. Still, this book closely aligns with the ruined past in Edensor's work, as he describes it: 'because of imperatives to bury the past too swiftly in search of the new, modernity is haunted in a particularly urgent fashion by that which has been consigned to irrelevance but which demands recognition of its historical impact' (2005, 830). Indeed, much of this book has sought to uncover the links between the frayed histories of the past and the impulse toward modernity, stability, and wellness. There is, additionally, a way to see ruins as analogous to sickness; that is, in their proximity to decay and disrepair, ruins stand in contrast to the complete, stable, and robust appearance that we have often ascribed to modernity. The able-bodied among us imagine ourselves in much the same way: we are moving forward, healthy and sure, and we rarely imagine the state of decay that we move toward.

Most of us order our lives and the spaces we inhabit around fullness and health, be it the health or wellbeing of a building or site, a body or mind, or a space and its history. In this book, I have argued that an emerging sense of feeling sick by and around people with HIV/AIDS in the 1980s shifted cultural perceptions of a host of things: sex, perceptions of risk and risky practices, bodily health, history, and cultural mores. The concomitant sense of feeling healthy prior to the HIV/AIDS pandemic similarly organized a prevailing worldview that affected our interactions with others and the world in which we live. To shift the focus by inspecting the ruins and sickly spaces around us is another way of feeling sickness, a necessary move that pays attention to the crumbling infrastructures we all inhabit.

Noting just how varied the practices of fixing memory to spaces are, Edensor nevertheless argues that 'there are undoubtedly tendencies to fix authoritative meanings about the past through an ensemble of practices and technologies which centre upon the production of specific spaces, here identified as monumental "memoryscapes"—mediated spaces, heritage districts, and museums' (2005, 530). For Edensor, such memoryscapes (in much the same way as Pierre Nora's 'sites of memory' or Christine Boyer's 'rhetorical topoi') organize national relationships with the past, are reified and mediatized, produce 'historic' districts through the conservation and gentrification of older spaces, and set forth specific narratives that seek to capture the idea of a period through narrative and dramatization (2005, 830–31). By focusing on ruins as disorderly sites of memory, Edensor looks to thwart the danger that the aforementioned 'regulated, commodified, highly encoded, desensualised sites of memory might become all-pervasive in the spatialization of memory' (2005, 833). The commodification of memory, in turn, is precisely a danger because it risks creating monoliths of memoryscapes wherein the past and its memory are linked to one select truth, as has been done with HIV/AIDS since the early years of the epidemic. Such selective forgetting and remembering solidifies 'the idea that there are places for remembering and places where memories and the past are irrelevant' (Edensor 2005, 833).

Nothing seems more irrelevant than ruins, places of rust and decay. They resist neat packaging attempts to relegate meaning to set districts or neighborhoods, and they are messy and chaotic, crumbling eyesores that stand out against the ordered nature of contemporary spaces. Yet, as Samuel Amago writes, 'the abandoned and decaying place has always fascinated the modern imaginary' (2019, 150). Such a fascination appears in Romantic and modernist works, Amago notes, as well as in Spanish realist novels of the late nineteenth century, 'where wasted spaces begin to appear more clearly as products of the growing hegemony of liberal capitalist modernity' (2019, 150). Edensor, in turn, asserts that ruins are 'replete with excess matter, including numerous obscure traces, [and] they are particularly charged by multiple yet elusive memories, as insubstantial as the ghosts who haunt them' (2005, 834). That excess matter can look like many things: discarded bottles or drug paraphernalia, fragmented shards of glass, multi-hued layers of paint peeling back from a wall, bricks with barely discernible letters written on them, and more. Outside of artistic production, it seems that we mostly look at these things as messy distractions from memory—proof of a past of some sort, but not one that matters. We think of ruins as little more than detritus, or someone's garbage.[1]

I want to return briefly to that first ruin, las Escuelas Pías de San Fernando. It was, of course, part of a string of purportedly 'ruined' spaces in Madrid at the time, sites that had been something else, had fallen into disuse and disrepair, and were repurposed over the ensuing decades. Constructed

1 Much of what I am arguing here has links with a host of works in Spanish urban studies, and particularly with those that study urban ecologies in Spain. I see these connections as emerging from the profound ties that health and environment have, which is to say that so much of how and where we live affects our health and wellbeing. Interested readers should refer to Amago (2021), Larson (2021), and Prádanos (2018), as well as the Hispanic Urban Studies edited series by Fraser and Larson through Palgrave Macmillan. Unlike these works, however, my focus is ultimately on illness and the politics of the ruin; that is, the political and physical collapse of spaces that was intimately tied to the physical deterioration expected of the person with AIDS at this time.

between 1763 and 1791, the area where the church and parochial school sat was around the size of a modern-day city block, bordered by the streets Mesón de Paredes to the east, Tribulete to the south, Embajadores and the Mercado de San Fernando to the west, and the Plaza de Agustín Lara to the north. The church, which functioned as such for hundreds of years, was burned down in 1936 during the Spanish Civil War, and only parts of the compound were rehabilitated over the ensuing decades. In fact, the abandoned and hollowed-out parts of the church in large part account for the dangerous ruins described in news articles by Sánchez and others during this period. In 1977, the largest section of the ruined church (on Mesón de Paredes) was declared a 'Monumento Nacional' 'a carácter de vestigio ejemplo del estilo protobarroco italiano del siglo XVII' (Herranz Durández 2016, 8). The status of 'Monumento Nacional', retitled to 'Bien de Interés Cultural' in 1985, is meant to afford the highest protection possible to the structure in question. Despite this designation, the Escuelas Pías de San Fernando was allowed to crumble further into disrepair and alternative use by those without homes, drug users, and others who had been relegated to the margins of society.

While the church decayed and deteriorated over the decades, adjacent areas experienced flashes of resurgence. The part of the site on Tribulete that had previously housed the parochial school of San Fernando was converted into a cinema, Cine Lavapiés, with a cabaret, the famous Molino Rojo (1955–1983), in the basement under it. When the cinema closed, this part of the Escuelas Pías also briefly housed the Teatro Lavapiés for a short period of years (roughly 1979–1984). In 1987, the building passed into the hands of the municipal government. It was rather unceremoniously and abruptly torn down in 1993, with the local government citing subsidence damage to the foundations and primary architectural structures of the building. The open lot sat abandoned for several years until 1996, when the Escuelas Pías was redesignated as 'Bien de Interés Cultural'; in 1998, the municipal government approved the UNED's use of the space, though the neighboring nave and church itself were not rehabilitated until 2002, when the UNED converted it into their library.

This brief history of the Escuelas Pías and the area surrounding it hints at any number of stories and memories, though its official history tends to skip over its disrepair, its occupation and notoriety in the 1980s, and the incongruous histories of sex, nightlife, and drugs that buffet the pristine images of church-become-library. The UNED redesign and conversion in 2000 silenced many of those micro-histories in favor of a much smoother narrative that aligns the spirit and the mind in esoteric harmony: it was a church, it was destroyed in the civil war, and it has been converted into a library. In this way, and though the Escuelas Pías does not fall into the precise type of ruin he describes, I see much in common with Edensor's descriptions of how we perceive industrial ruins. He writes:

> Whereas classical and romantic ruins are primarily apprehended by the gaze, the sensual experience of moving inside a ruin is characterized by immanent immersion rather than by a scopic, distanced sensing, seduced by the symbolic and aesthetic placings of ornaments and images. The tactilities of ruins are characterized by matter crumbling underfoot, the crunch of mortar and broken glass, and the feel of decaying matter. The body is apt to be buffeted by wind and rain, by gusts heavy with dust, and by atmospheres thick with the presence of damp. The relatively quiescent soundscape becomes a composite of lower-decibel murmurs, soft echoes, and scurries of unseen movement: the drips of water, eddies of winds, creaking machinery and doors, the cooing of pigeons and their flurries of urgent flight. Similarly, ruined smellscapes are a heady brew of damp masonry, rotting wood and fungus, acrid chemicals, and the surprising bouquets of summer flowers. (2005, 837–38)

Edensor is purposefully offering a sensorially rich and pleasing cluster of sensations, sights, and smells in order to combat the reputation of ruins as lifeless, decayed, and dirty. Reading past the poetics, we can see a distinction between types of ruins and the experiences they offer to visitors; that is, the industrial ruin is not a place by which one might be visually seduced, but an unseemly space in actual decay. This description seems aptly to describe the state of the Escuelas Pías in its years of decline, despite it pointedly not being an industrial ruin. As the concerned neighbors in 'Vecinos de Embajadores...' recount it: 'Hemos hecho lo que tenía que haber hecho la Policía. Ellos no han podido y lo hemos hecho nosotros, pero aquello no fue un acto violento: solo quemamos basura' [We have done what the police should have done. They weren't able to and we did it, but it was not a violent act: we only burned garbage] (Sánchez 1985, 43). By underscoring its actions as non-violent because they only involved detritus—as opposed to the actions of the itinerant occupants of the ruined church, who are unanimously blamed for the uptick in violent attacks around the neighborhood—the group effectively localizes crime to ruins and associates those criminals and their effects with refuse. The romantic notion of the church's value (i.e., its historical importance) is of little significance to the neighborhood residents, who only see its decay, disrepair, and repurposed use as a shelter for illicit acts.

This is not to downplay the actual crime rate or the swollen numbers of intravenous drug users in the area, which were rampant in the early years of the 1980s; nor is this critique meant to understate the frustration and fear that neighborhood associations and residents felt at this time. In fact, according to Francisco Fernández de Alba, there was broad distrust toward municipal governments at this time with regards to city planning and management. Writing on the state of Madrid in the earliest years of the Transition, Fernández de Alba comments how

> public debate on urbanism and the continuous stream of scandalous news about urban speculation and fraudulent construction deals had a measurable effect on Madrid residents ... They saw their city as a chaotic, dense agglomeration. They noted traffic problems and the lack of resources (schools, hospitals, cultural centres), and associated the evident physical decay of Madrid with its less tangible social decline. (2020, 27–28)

Such evident physical decay is corroborated by Duncan Wheeler, who notes that '70 per cent of properties in inner Madrid (calculated as being within the circumference of the M-30 ring-road) were classified as uninhabitable at the time of Franco's death' (2020, 190). As their lack of faith in newly elected officials grew, *madrileños* increasingly turned to neighborhood associations, which 'had grown in number and strength throughout the early seventies ... as a consequence of poor urban conditions and the lack of an effective municipal response' (Fernández de Alba 2020, 28). Though such associations would eventually link up into urban social movements and have a powerful say in the shape of the city in years to come, this early moment in the 1980s saw them still dealing with an inefficient and ineffective municipal government.

This is clearly seen in an article from *ABC* from 1983, 'Los vecinos de Arganzuela, hartos de robos y asaltos' [The residents of Arganzuela, fed up with robberies and assaults], which starts powerfully and forcefully by describing how the residents of the Arganzuela neighborhood deal with daily robberies, muggings, and sex workers lining their streets. The article draws particular attention to Tribulete, a street bordering Escuelas Pías that frequently appears in reports on crime in Embajadores.

> En la [calle] de Tribulete se ha cometido ahora un asesinato, pero la ola de delincuencia no es nueva en esta vía. Desde hace ya mucho tiempo, los asaltos a establecimientos y a transeúntes se dan cada dos por tres. Y, además, tienen que soportar cómo impunemente jóvenes de

> no muy buena reputación en la barriada y maleantes de la peor calaña se dedican a negociar en plena vía pública con la droga. El trapicheo de estupefacientes se puede comprobar incluso a plena luz del día. (D. 1983)[2]

Further on in the article, the author writes that 'en la plaza de Agustín Lara ... los jóvenes llegan a lavar en una fuente pública las jeringuillas con las que se acaban de inyectar "caballo" (heroína)' [in the Plaza de Agustín Lara ... young people come to wash the syringes with which they have injected 'smack' (heroin) in a public fountain] (D. 1983).[3] The image of Spanish youth washing out dirty needles in a public fountain is meant to be a grotesque one for the newspaper's readership, and it both recurs to and builds on a sense of physical and moral cleanliness and decorum. In this way, these articles (and many like them) tie together concepts of citizenship, goodness, and cleanliness with the urban spaces or ruins that one inhabits. These spaces are further linked to crime and drug use, a metonymic slide from physical ruins to ruined lives.

Crisis and crash

What does it mean to be seen continually as living a ruined life, or to occupy spaces that are always in ruin? One of the key concerns of this chapter is to understand the framing of HIV/AIDS among intravenous drug users in these early years, which was so often under a politics of the ruin; that is, a perception of life in shambles, in disrepair, and unable to be recovered. The political struggles that occurred around HIV/AIDS and drug use at this time were often attempts to recover lives, despite overwhelming social pressure and a cultural imaginary that saw particular people as lost causes. This had immense downstream consequences for local and state policies and initiatives as well as for people living with HIV/AIDS.

2 'A murder has been committed on Tribulete, but crime waves are not new on this street. For a while now, attacks on businesses and pedestrians have been happening all the time. And furthermore, [residents] have to endure how young people of ill repute and thugs of the worst kind make a living by dealing drugs out in the open with impunity. Drug dealing can be seen even in broad daylight.'

3 As discussed earlier, it is apparent that both *ABC* articles were looking to demonize those who used drugs in a number of ways, particularly when they are painted as outsiders to the area and connected to the rising drug culture among Spanish youth. This, of course, was in part because of the conservative nature and readership of *ABC* as a newspaper, but it also demonstrates just how drug use, drug users, and the ruined spaces they inhabited were framed at this time.

Previous chapters of this book have documented the origin narrative of AIDS in Spain through the lens of its first three known cases: an anonymous homosexual man in Barcelona in 1981 and two young boys with hemophilia in Sevilla in 1983 and 1984. Moving through their histories, I discussed how queerness, illness, and innocence became entangled alongside the political and social repercussions of this narrative. Though concepts of illegality and risk are shot through the way HIV/AIDS was discussed at this time, intravenous drug users remained the recalcitrant risk takers in this narrative, and were often portrayed as unreformable and discardable in popular culture and news. This narrative has also been seen in the statements and actions of some Embajadores neighborhood associations at the time, which portray drug use as external and non-local, belonging to a ruined space that lies outside of the social and municipal borders of citizenry.

Juan Carlos Usó, who has written a number of foundational studies on drugs in Spanish culture, relates the search for identity to the influx of drugs into Spain. Citing the effects of the economic crisis of 1973, Usó writes that young people were forced to confront the realities of day-to-day living even in the midst of monumental political change: 'El *punk* y la sensación de no-futuro impactó entre las primeras generaciones de la transición, desplazando las ansias psiquedélicas. Otras drogas, como la heroína, iban a reaparecer con fuerza en la escena española' [Punk and the sense of no future impacted the first generations of the Transition, displacing their thirst for psychedelics. Other drugs, such as heroin, were poised to make a strong comeback on the Spanish scene] (1996, 287). Noting 'a certain overlap' between the policies of Francoist and transitional Spain (2020, 69), Fernández de Alba builds on the work done by Usó by critiquing the representation of drugs at the time, as distinct from actual drug use and drug culture. Such a differentiation is crucial, as it recognizes that the most common portrayals of drug use in this period do not always (or often) capture the whole picture. To this point, Fernández de Alba writes that the uptick in substance abuse in the late 1970s and early 1980s in Spain 'occurred against the backdrop of profound economic transformation characterized by a move from an agrarian, deeply Catholic, moralistic, vertically integrated authoritarian society to a liberal, post-industrial, increasingly secular, democratic consumer society' (2020, 76). In Tom Whittaker's extensive consideration of these changes in his work on the Spanish *quinqui* film, he critiques the fact that 'the threadbare state overseen by Franco spectacularly failed to shield the weakest in society from economic fallout. Despite its recent economic fortunes, the regime had maintained a very low expenditure on welfare services and social investment' (2020, 3). The resulting effect saw a corresponding rise in crime rates, as Whittaker notes, citing an 87.59% increase in burglaries and a 100% rise in vehicle theft between 1975 and 1979, which were often attributed to teenage delinquency (2020, 3). Like Usó, Fernández de Alba and Whittaker see the increase in drug use and domestic crime in Spain as part of the political moment, an eruption tied to the monumental political shift the country faced as it transitioned to democracy.

The promise of political change in the Transition, along with the concurrent opening of new markets and routes of commerce and a dizzying sense of freedom, formed a potent cocktail. From cocaine to hashish to heroin, drug use soared in Spain in the late 1970s and through the 1980s, with differing meanings for the increasing numbers of Spaniards who chose to partake. This is to say that, for many, drug use was a form of experimentation and a means to express identity, but it also became a dangerous and wasting addiction. The most dangerous and deadly of these drugs was heroin, the use of which soon reached epidemic proportions. As Whittaker relays, in the early 1980s 'a famous military figure had commented that heroin had now overtaken terrorism as the most serious problem in Spain' (2020, 121). In his study on heroin use in Spain, Juan F. Gamella calls the heroin crisis 'una forma de politoxicomanía centrada alrededor del consume habitual y compulsivo de heroína, sobre todo por vía intravenosa, que en unos años se extendió masivamente, hasta convertirse en un problema de salud pública y de control social, mayoritariamente percibido como tal por la población' [a form of multi-drug addiction centered around the habitual and compulsive consumption of heroin, especially intravenously, which in a few years spread massively until it became a problem of public health and social control, mostly perceived as such by the population] (1997, 20). What exactly gave rise to the proliferation of heroin use is still debated, though there are some commonalities across studies: namely, a sense of freedom of expression and identity, as we have already seen, and increasing availability of the drug.

Gamella, looking to the first medical reports of heroin users in Spain, narrows the rise in usage to the early years of the Transition and notes that in the summer of 1978 one could still count heroin users by the dozens, while in 1982 'había ya en España decenas de miles de jóvenes que había aprendido a inyectarse opiáceos que conseguían en un creciente mercado negro, y que se consideraban a sí mismos adictos a la heroína' [there were already tens of thousands of young people in Spain who had learned to inject opiates obtained from a growing black market, and who were considered addicted to heroin] (1997, 22). Like nearly all other scholars of drug use in Spain at this time, Gamella sees the late 1970s and early 1980s as crucial in the Spanish heroin crisis. He divides the years into various critical 'phases' of the heroin epidemic: 1977–1978, when the first addicts become visible to the public; 1979–1982, when drug use reached epidemic levels; and a third phase in 1983–1986, the true zenith of drug use, when there was a definitive institutionalization of the problem. From 1987 onward, according to Gamella, the crisis entered a new/final phase, in which the number of new users diminished even as morbidity and mortality among them rose. In this final phase, heroin was more commonly smoked (and mixed with cocaine), which was seen as less dangerous than intravenous injection (Gamella 1997, 22).

As heroin usage grew, so too did its clear and debilitating effects on public health. Gamella sums up heroin's troubling effects on one's body by noting how 'inyectarse en vena varias veces al día sustancias adulteradas y contaminadas, con poca higiene y control de las inyecciones ya supone por sí solo un considerable riesgo para la salud' [injecting adulterated and contaminated substances into a vein several times a day, with poor hygiene and control, already poses a considerable risk to health by itself] (1997, 26). Beyond that, heroin users found themselves visited with a host of other illnesses and health issues: hepatitis, tuberculosis, endocarditis, as well as embolisms, gangrene, abscesses, and much more (1997, 26). These effects often tend to snowball, says Gamella, who continues by asserting that 'el desprecio de sí que suele acompañar a esa dependencia conduce a muchos heroinómanos al abandono y la falta de interés y cuidado en su alimentación, higiene, etcétera, lo que incide también en la morbilidad de este colectivo' [the self-contempt that usually accompanies this dependence leads many heroin addicts to neglect, and lack of interest and care in their diet, hygiene, etc., which also affects the morbidity of this group] (1997, 26).

The picture that emerges is that of a country coming out of a dictatorship and freewheeling headfirst into rampant drug use. In the case of heroin, what appeared to begin as a marker of status and libertine enjoyment quickly spread through the population and to young people of all economic backgrounds; affecting working-class and poor youth disproportionately, intravenous heroin use eventually contributed to rising delinquency in Spain while causing breakdowns in public health and safety. At the same time, and just as intravenous drug use began to spread and take hold in the youth population, the HIV epidemic exploded in Spain.

A tale of two Hs: Heroin and HIV

Some years into what would become a heroin crisis—and two years into an encroaching AIDS epidemic—a 1983 issue of the medical journal *Medicina Clínica* detailed one of the first diagnosed cases in Spain among drug users. As the authors write, 'hasta la actualidad solo cuatro pacientes residentes en España han sido diagnosticados de este síndrome, un varón homosexual y tres pacientes hemofílicos. Recientemente hemos tenido ocasión de diagnosticar un nuevo caso de SIDA en un varón toxicómano con relaciones homosexuales esporádicas, residente en Barcelona' [To date, only four patients residing in Spain have been diagnosed with this syndrome, one homosexual man and three hemophiliacs. We have recently had the opportunity to diagnose a new case of AIDS in a male drug addict with sporadic homosexual relationships, living in Barcelona] (Estruch et al. 1983, 645). As seen in the earlier descriptions of the first few cases of HIV/AIDS in Spain, this article goes to some lengths to list all the possible suspicious avenues of contagion, stating that

> se trata de un varón de 18 años de edad que fue estudiado en mayo de 1983 por presentar desde hacia 18 meses fiebre diaria de 38° C, astenia, pérdida de 16 kg de peso y poliadenopatías. El paciente era adicto a la heroína intravenosa desde hacia tres años y utilizaba para su administración el mismo material que un homosexual con el que además mantenía relaciones sexuales esporádicas (una o dos al mes) y que en junio de 1981 había visitado Nueva York. (Estruch et al. 1983, 645)[4]

The authors additionally note that the young man had been diagnosed with hepatitis B nearly a year earlier and a severe ear infection three months earlier, details which establish a vague but damning history of sickness. The entirety of this medical narrative suggests a past of bad habits and infectious acts by this anonymous man—not only in his heroin use but in his sporadic trysts with a man who had visited New York in 1981, a dubious move intended to epidemiologically maintain HIV/AIDS as a foreign illness. This second man returns to the narrative later, his story fleshed out as that of 'un homosexual que había mantenido relaciones con otros homosexuales neoyorquinos en 1981' [a homosexual who had sexual relationships with other New York homosexuals in 1981] (Estruch et al. 1983, 645). This information might be interpreted as a sort of contact tracing or a cursory way to underscore the origins and spread of the patient's illness, but it clearly scapegoats homosexuals and perceptions of urban queer spaces in the United States as particularly riddled with AIDS. In this manner, and rather than interrogate too deeply the paths of HIV infection and transmission in

4 'This is an 18-year-old male who was studied in May 1983 for having a daily fever of 38° C for about 18 months, asthenia, weight loss of 16 kg, and polyadenopathy. The patient had been addicted to intravenous heroin for three years and used the same paraphernalia as a homosexual with whom he also had sporadic sexual relations (once or twice a month) and who in June 1981 had visited New York.'

Spain, the physicians in this case settle for a type of shorthand that blames foreign homosexuals as the root cause of AIDS.

More clearly than in the earlier cases discussed in Chapter 1, the long-term (18-month) fever connected to this man's illness suggests that he had presented symptoms associated with HIV for the better part of a year, which could place his seroconversion anywhere from late 1981 to the earlier half of 1982. I note this not as an attempt to pinpoint a precise date for the man's illness but to show how out of sorts the timeline for HIV/AIDS has always been, whether in Spain or elsewhere. To put it simply: the idea that Spain was immune to the spread of HIV/AIDS, or even that AIDS was not present in the population until some years after it appeared the United States, is not at all accurate. We see once again, then, how HIV/AIDS went untreated, undiagnosed, and unheard of for at least a couple of years, if not longer. This fact was not entirely lost on the authors of the article, who recall the earlier diagnosis of the anonymous homosexual man in 1981 recounted in Chapter 1, noting how his symptoms emerged 'coetáneamente con el inicio del cuadro clínico de nuestro paciente' [contemporaneously with the onset of our patient's clinical signs] (Estruch et al. 1983, 645). Placing these two cases in the same orbit produces a nagging worry for the doctors that 'junto a la detección de otros dos nuevos casos que estamos estudiando en la actualidad, nos hacen sospechar un aumento en los próximos meses en el número de pacientes afectos de SIDA en nuestro medio' [together with the detection of two other new cases that we are currently studying, this makes us suspect an increase in the coming months in the number of patients with AIDS in our surroundings] (Estruch et al. 1983, 645). Though not given much thought in this article beyond its mention, the chronology here allows for a fuller understanding of HIV transmission in Spain. That is, beyond the immediate fear of a catastrophic rise in cases, the simultaneity of the anonymous homosexual discussed in Chapter 1 and this heroin user underscores a fact not regularly considered in public origin narratives of illness, which is that initial contact points of infection are most often multiple and varied, occurring through a range of means and groups. This is to say that it is entirely feasible—indeed, highly likely—that HIV entered Spain through men who had sex with men, through blood product, and through intravenous drug use at the same time, spreading in a parallel fashion through varied avenues and communities that did not necessarily have frequent contact with each other.

To be clear, this was perhaps not entirely obvious in the middle of the pandemic, when medical professionals, journalists, and government institutions were all scrambling to provide a context for an unfolding health crisis. It is, however, revealing to see what or who gets emphasized and scapegoated in these early years. A 1986 report from the *Morbidity and Mortality Weekly Report* (*MMWR*) of the Centers for Disease Control and Prevention makes clear just how virulent this outbreak narrative had become in Spain, particularly against the backdrop of reported AIDS cases. The report notes that of the 1,330 European patients with HIV/AIDS reported to the World Health Organization,

> 1,031 (78%) were homosexual or bisexual. Ninety (7%) patients were IV drug abusers, and 21 (2%), both homosexual and IV drug abusers. These 111 cases were diagnosed in: Italy—45; Spain—26; the Federal Republic of Germany—14; France—11; Switzerland—seven; Austria—four; the United Kingdom—three; and Sweden—one. Fifty-two (4%) of the reported patients had hemophilia and were diagnosed in: the Federal Republic of Germany—21; Spain—12; the United Kingdom—nine; France—three; Sweden—two; and one each in Austria, Denmark, Greece, Italy, and Norway. (Centers for Disease Control and Prevention 1986)

I cite the full data in this section to give a sense of Spain's numbers when compared to those of other European countries. This is perhaps not an entirely fair comparison, as the *MMWR* report itself notes, due to 'differences that may exist in the methods of data collection' or the fact that 'in countries where AIDS is still rare, distribution may be modified with the increase in number of cases' (Centers for Disease Control and Prevention 1986). It is nevertheless useful to see that with regards to hemophiliacs and IV drug users, the numbers in Spain are the second highest; it is also important contextualization to note that while male homosexual HIV/AIDS cases 'accounted for 60%–100% of the total number of cases in 12 of 16 countries' (Centers for Disease Control and Prevention 1986), this was not the case in Spain. Alongside Belgium, Greece, and Italy, gay men accounted for less than 50% of HIV/AIDS cases. What becomes apparent, again, is just how much the AIDS health crisis (in Spain and beyond) was at once manifold and unconstrained to any one group. It also becomes increasingly clear that the focus on any one purported risk group always came at the cost of Spanish lives, and that the spread of HIV/AIDS has never been limited to those groups that were deemed particularly viral by an established outbreak narrative.

This story is infrequently told. Examining the earliest known cases of HIV/AIDS in the 1980s, as shown in the first chapter, in fact demonstrates how carefully constructed the origin narrative was for the epidemic, and how frequently homosexuals and drug users were seen as the originators and key cause of HIV transmission. A combination of scientific fact and magical thinking, the origin story of AIDS was predicated on moral panic, homophobia, and a sense of insulated security, among many other things. What it left out was just as important and often went unspoken, half spoken, or only hazily sketched out. Despite data that suggested otherwise, in the origin story of HIV/AIDS in Spain, the figure of the infected drug user served as this ghostly presence, one who appears contemporaneously alongside the anonymous gay man of 1981 or the hemophiliac brothers in Sevilla but who receives even shorter shrift, not so much a person but an *idea* of one, made to stand in for a whole class of ruined lives and people.

No way out: Inside the prison

Though the concept of guilt and innocence has been intentionally complicated throughout this book as is the porousness of the risk groups of AIDS, which were often blended and mutable—early reports spent a great deal of effort in sorting communities by their perceived dangerousness and guilt. This approach has been clearly shown throughout this book, most notably in news reports from the early 1980s in Spain. In one such report, 'Cárceles: Miedo al SIDA' (August 3, 1986), the news program *El Dominical* turned to the dramatic increases in cases of HIV seen in the prison population in Spain. The report opens with an anonymous prisoner speaking of the relationship between drugs and life in prison, reporting that

> se trata por todos los medios de conseguir la droga al precio que sea, como sea, no importa la forma que te vayas a meter la heroína o te vayas a meter lo que te vayas a meter, una pastilla machacada, lo que sea ... Entonces coges cualquier jeringuilla, no te importa de donde viene ... Si viene de una enfermedad, de una infección, o de una gente que tiene los principios de SIDA, o que tienen contagio—eso, enfermedad—y te lo metes de la forma que puedes. ('Cárceles: Miedo al SIDA' 1986)[5]

The blinding need of addiction—whether in a prison or outside of it—leads the addict to increasingly risky actions. In the enclosed ecosystem of the prison, these risky actions are amplified and can result in an uncontrolled outbreak. What's more, and as the host of the report states, the prison

5 'It's about getting the drug by all means and at whatever price, however you can, no matter how you are going to take the heroin or whatever you're going to take, a crushed pill, whatever ... Then you grab any syringe, you don't care where it comes from ... If it comes from a disease, an infection, or somebody who's got the beginnings of AIDS, or with some kind of contagion—whatever, illness—and you take it any way you can.'

hospital 'añade a las dificultades de una institución penitenciaria las derivadas de la atención de un amplio número de enfermedades. Aquí el paciente, además de estar enfermo, está preso, y por lo tanto sometido a las imposiciones de un régimen carcelario' [adds the difficulty of caring for a large number of sick to the difficulties of running a penitentiary. Here, the patient is incarcerated in addition to being sick, and therefore subjected to the impositions of a prison regime] ('Cárceles: Miedo al SIDA' 1986). As the voiceover explains, in this space, the addict or the sick person is never only these things—he is also a prisoner who must bear the punitive weight of the legal system to which he is indebted.

In their article 'AIDS and the Prison System', Dubler and Sidel frame this as a formal problem with the very structure of the prison itself: 'Prisons are confining, not caring, institutions, and adapting to AIDS presents a fundamental dilemma. Their responses lay bare discrepancies between social expectations about the "correctional" function of prisons and the reality' (1991, 71). The authors go on to note how efforts to cope with disease further amplify the debate about what healthcare in prison can even look like, particularly in a system that in most cases is only designed to be punitive (1991, 71). To be clear, the perennial problem of care within a punitive system was not addressed in these early years of AIDS in Spain, at least not satisfactorily. Despite a lead time of several years between the first known intravenous drug users with HIV and the interviews with prisoners in the news report, there is still a chasm between knowledge and preventive action. As a prisoner in 'Cárceles: Miedo al SIDA' grimly explains,

> Hay una psicosis generalizada de la gente por el peligro del SIDA, ¿no? Ya que te traen a gente que está por aquí también con el SIDA. La gente, pues, en fin, no hay ninguna medida aquí contra ellos, ¿no? Ni nos tienen informados para prevención de esto ni—en fin, se puede coger aquí infinidad de enfermedades. ('Cárceles: Miedo al SIDA' 1986)[6]

Whether intentionally or not, the 'infinite' possibilities of illness in prison function directly in service of the prison as a place of punishment. This is to say that all illness—but the particularly dark specter of HIV/AIDS at this time—becomes another tool of torture and punishment in prison.

In the most generous of readings, the weaponization of HIV and AIDS in the prison system was accidental, and its spread was only the product of

6 'There is a generalized psychosis of people because of the danger of AIDS, right? Since they bring in people around here who also have AIDS. These people, well, there isn't any measure taken here against them, right? They don't advise us on how to prevent this or—anyways, you can catch an infinity of diseases here.'

confinement, boredom, and basic human desires for tactility and pleasure. Once HIV/AIDS was introduced into prison populations, however, death was often seen as a *fait accompli.* So whether it was accidental, wished for, or planned, the rapid rate of infection was rarely inhibited in the early years of the epidemic. In the *El Dominical* report discussed above, HIV is in fact portrayed not as a possibility but as a terrifying inevitability. In one particular sequence, prisoners are shown entering their cells, slowly walking up a flight of stairs accompanied by dark, non-diegetic marching music. A narrator's bleak message accompanies this sequence: 'La droga es un problema que lleva sus consecuencias más allá de las originadas directamente por los alucinógenos. Generado en ocasiones por el uso de jeringuillas ya utilizadas, el ritmo de contagio del SIDA parece, de momento, imparable' [Drugs are a problem that carries consequences beyond those caused directly by hallucinogens. Sometimes generated by the use of already-used syringes, the rate of contagion of AIDS seems, for the moment, unstoppable] ('Cárceles: Miedo al SIDA' 1986). Matching the rhythmic music to the rate or 'rhythm' of contagion of AIDS, the prisoners are seen to be on a death march, alive but already dead and dying in the liminality of illness.

The perception of HIV/AIDS in the prison system as an ever present inevitability was brought about and fueled by what Rut Martín Hernández has called 'pasotismo institucional' (2009, 248), a term that adequately describes the institutional-level apathy in prison with regards to the life, health, and wellbeing of its constituents. Martín Hernández further decries the penal institution itself, saying that 'se ignora el hecho de que muchos presos consumen drogas por vía intravenosa convirtiendo estas instituciones en lugares en los que la posibilidad de contagio es muy alta' [the fact that many prisoners consume drugs intravenously is ignored, turning these institutions into places where the possibility of contagion is very high], a problem that further buries any possible preventive campaign outreach (2009, 248). Though she is writing on the prison system of 2009, the message is the same: if the root cause of the problem (here, the fact of drug use in the prison population) can be made invisible or ignored, then there will be no need for cure or treatment.

Some of this institutional apathy is clearly at work in 'Cárceles: Miedo al SIDA' when Miguel Araña Romero, the medical director of a penitentiary hospital, explains that a patient's HIV diagnosis is kept in strict confidence from his inmates: 'El paciente, desde luego, que tiene un marcador positive lo conoce. Los otros, no. O si lo conocen, no somos nosotros los médicos los que se lo hemos comentado' [The seropositive patient, of course, knows it. Others do not. Or if they know it, it's not we doctors who have told them] ('Cárceles: Miedo al SIDA' 1986). Though argued differently by the inmates themselves, who fear the rampant spread of the virus and who develop justifiably paranoid reactions to others who are in prison with them, this part of Araña Romero's logic is somewhat understandable. He follows this, however, by dismissing the prisoners' concerns precisely because they are prisoners and drug users:

> De todas maneras, el [hecho de] que existan estas prácticas y el [hecho de] que exista un uso común de ciertas jeringas, pienso que no es labor de los médicos en cuanto a la vigilancia. Sí en cuanto al decirle al estamento regimental que estas cosas no deben ocurrir. Pero no deben ocurrir ni aquí ni en la calle. Quiero decir que no somos nosotros los que debemos de vigilar este uso. ('Cárceles: Miedo al SIDA' 1986)[7]

Perhaps in the strictest sense of his words, Araña Romero is right that it is not (or not chiefly) the responsibility of the medical professionals in prison to monitor, limit, or control the needle sharing or drug use of the inmates. This is, perhaps a generous reading of his meaning, which seems to shrug off responsibility out of a nihilistic outlook regarding the potential of treatment. That is, this statement implies that these men are only recalcitrant addicts and is likely further bolstered by the simplistic perception of them as criminals, as opposed to a multifaceted understanding of them as complex people. It is a view that flattens the person into nothing more than a sick criminal addict. And if this prisoner is going to use drugs regardless of where he is, and if drug use in and of itself is a danger or 'bad', then why bother?

An April 24, 1987, *La Vanguardia* editorial described the grim situation of the prison system in Spain primarily in reaction to such carceral logic and apathy. The editorial looks to the rolling outbreaks of HIV/AIDS in prison populations and considers just how unknown these numbers are: 'Si bien no se conoce con seguridad cuál es la proporción de reclusos que padece el mal, los entendidos estiman que aumenta constantemente, y mientras unos aseguran que pasa de la mitad, otros llegan a estimar que en algunos centros ronda el 70 por ciento' [Although the percentage of inmates suffering from the disease is not known with certainty, experts estimate that it is constantly increasing, and while some claim that it exceeds half, others estimate that in some centers it is around 70%] (*La Vanguardia*

7 'In any case, the [fact that] these practices exist and [that] there is common use of certain syringes, I think that surveillance is not the job of physicians. Sure, we should tell the establishment that these things shouldn't happen. But they shouldn't happen here or on the street. I mean that we are not the ones who should monitor this use.'

1987). There is a chance that these figures are inflated, but underreporting, misdiagnosis, institutional apathy, and lack of preventative treatment would most certainly allow for the rampant spread of illness in this manner. Placing the estimated figures up against the prison population, the editorial asks whether capital punishment—here, death from complications from HIV/AIDS—is proportionate to the crime. It notes that, near the time of its writing, there were

> unas veinticinco mil personas en las prisiones españoles. Veinticuatro mil hombres y unas mil trescientas mujeres. El setenta por ciento largo de los que están en la cárcel han entrado en ella antes de los treinta años por delitos que en sesenta y seis por ciento de los casos son contra la propiedad. Las cárceles custodian tanto a los detenidos, los presos preventivos que esperan, a veces durante mucho tiempo, juicio, como a los penados que cumplen condena. Son menos de noventa establecimientos penitenciarios, la mitad de ellos instalados en edificios antiguos. (*La Vanguardia* 1987)[8]

This account goes against the popular imaginary of a prison as filled with only the most hardened and lifelong criminals; instead, the editorial reminds the reader that a prison holds those who are waiting for sentencing, those who have only been arrested but not yet charged, those who have committed minor infractions, and the relatively young. It also obliquely critiques the state of the prisons themselves. Its description of Spanish prisons as being housed in 'old buildings' offers a sense of the entire system itself as flawed, crumbling, derelict. Like the drug dens that notoriously spotted certain urban areas around Spain (Lavapiés and La Latina in Madrid, for example, or el Raval in Barcelona), the prison is portrayed as being in a metaphysical and literal state of disrepair. Unlike the Escuelas Pías, though, the prison and its system are not quite ruined just yet, though here they are seen as sites in the process of becoming ruins. That is, the figures and images paint a grim picture of uncontrolled and unchecked drug use in the prison system in Spain, a practice that leads to HIV/AIDS outbreaks; these outbreaks, in turn, are seen as a fitting punishment for deviance, in line with a broader social narrative about the illness. In this manner, lawlessness and illness

8 '[There are] some 25,000 people in Spanish prisons: 24,000 men and about 1300 women. Well over 70% of those who are in jail entered before the age of 30 for crimes that in 66% of cases were against property. Prisons hold those who have been arrested, detainees who wait (sometimes for a long time) for trial, as well as convicts who are serving their sentences. There are less than ninety prisons, half of them located in old buildings.'

twin together and are allowed to run rampant, while an institutional apathy toward the wellbeing of the imprisoned means that everything, from systems to physical spaces, crumbles all around them.

Under this logic, it is not a huge leap to think of the ruin as definitional in the understanding of HIV/AIDS, particularly in the case of seropositive intravenous drug users or prisoners. The same bellicose metaphors that are so often applied to illnesses, and which Sontag described so forcefully in her work, leave rubble and ruin in their wake. To speak of the ravages of illness, a body that fights and succumbs to AIDS, or the battle against drug addiction and institutional apathy is a way of describing a war in which there are casualties and losses. The prevalence of this descriptive language means we see illness as an enemy combatant; the unknowability of AIDS in the 1980s meant that cultural narratives and institutions also dreamed up sleeper agents, irrecoverable prisoners of war, and saw some populations and groups as sacrificial cannon fodder. None of this bellicose metaphorization is particularly novel, neither at the time that Sontag wrote nor in the decades since, but it leaves behind a mark. Or more specifically, it leaves behind ruins.

If we must cling to the war metaphors of illness—and there appears to be little sign of that changing—we must acknowledge what is left behind in the wake. In this case, we have the intersection of three ruined and ruinous figures: the intravenous drug user, who has been disregarded and maligned as both a ghost in the story of HIV/AIDS and one of its prime culprits; the person with AIDS, who faced a host of fatal possibilities in the early years of the epidemic; and the literal and figurative space of the prison, an institution that struggled to modernize and adapt to an ongoing public health crisis. In the first half of this chapter, I pointed to the shifting perceptions of drug use in Spain, how heroin became wrapped up into the unfolding health crisis of HIV/AIDS in the early 1980s, and the perception of addicts with AIDS in the prison system. Their stories are intertwined not only because an outbreak narrative forced them together, but because of a joint perception of these things as equally ruined, as detritus. What does it mean for the imprisoned drug user with HIV to be triply seen as ruined? Edensor sees the ruin as a space that is fundamentally haunted, and Amago describes the temporal nature of our relationships with ruins. Perhaps we see something of both here, not in an obvious or facile way, but in the sense that we have a figure, space, and illness that are neglected, made invisible, and allowed to fall into states of disrepair and exile from the larger community. The language we have available to us—wartime words and metaphors—and an ongoing search for expressing what AIDS actually *means* in this moment only secure its place as an edifice sliding into disrepair.

Carabanchel, crumbling

In the story of the Escuelas Pías, the development, deterioration, and eventual renovation of its buildings mirrors the story of betterment and self-repair that we demand from the down-and-out. The ruins and derelict, crumbling structures that became drug dens and refuges for those without homes are swept clean and upgraded, while their occupants are dispersed cleanly and quickly. We do not hear from them again—at least, not in the way that they were or are, but as new and improved versions of themselves. This does not always happen, of course; sometimes, ruins stay ruined, and a person or a group of people is dismissed as hopelessly lost. Some of this is at work in the stories of the people with HIV/AIDS at this time, and perhaps more so for those who were addicted to intravenous drugs.

The prison of Carabanchel, unlike the Escuelas Pías, does not have a particularly noble origin story or redemptive arc, though it underwent some of the same transformations that the crumbling ruins of Escuelas Pías saw. Its connections to lawlessness and crime, drugs and HIV make it a compelling counterpart to Escuelas Pías, though, in that they were both spaces that housed illness and crumbled around their occupants. Despite these commonalities, the prison is not—or perhaps cannot be—redeemed from its past. Located in the southwestern Madrid suburb of the same name, Carabanchel Prison was built from 1940 to 1944 during the dictatorship of Francisco Franco by political prisoners of the regime. The prison went through a number of phases: by the late 1970s, it was characterized by widespread riots led by the Coordinadora de Presos en Lucha (COPEL), a group of the imprisoned who fought for greater civil rights. Only a few years later, Carabanchel became even more infamous for its derelict condition, rampant drug use, and an unceasing HIV/AIDS problem. The prison was eventually closed in 1998, and the remaining inmates were sent to various other prisons. After a long period of debate about the afterlife of the abandoned complex, during which it decayed further and was occupied by a host of legal and extralegal entities, it was ultimately demolished in 2008. Over a decade later, the space where Carabanchel once was remains vacant.

This brief history of Carabanchel shows a continued state of decline and eventual collapse that began in the late 1970s and continued onward. In this tale of decline, the specter of illness is omnipresent, and there is no doubt that the spread of HIV/AIDS in the prison in the 1980s contributed to its reputation as being particularly gruesome. In their history of Carabanchel Prison, for example, Alfredo González-Ruibal and Carmen Ortiz write that it 'has been one of the most monumental and recognizable symbols of repression in Spain from its construction in 1940 until its destruction in 2008. Even today, it looms large in the imagination of many Spaniards as the quintessential space of punishment in the recent history of the country' (2015, 1). A symbol of Francoist repression and layered with decades of suffering, Carabanchel is a painful site of memory for many. This was no doubt compounded by the imposing structure of the building itself, with its panopticon of buildings that were clearly visible and towered over the Madrid neighborhoods of Carabanchel and Aluche (Ortiz García and Martínez Zauner 2016, 5).

Its latter years are of particular note here, when the building itself began to crumble, the prison conditions plumbed new depths, and when HIV/AIDS became an existential threat to the populace. The memory of Carabanchel in ruins is visible in numerous news articles that decry the prison conditions as well as televised reports from inside, like 'Cárceles: Miedo al SIDA'. One particular documentary, *Carabanchel: la otra orilla* (1987), was notable for its access and portrayal of the conditions in the prison at a time when HIV/AIDS was only just beginning to be understood by the larger populace. The documentary shows the catastrophic ruin that the prison had become, as well as the hopelessness and pain of the people inside it.

Carabanchel: la otra orilla was produced by Tele Prisión, a prison television network created, broadcast, and maintained by prisoners in Carabanchel from 1985 to 1987. The co-creator of Tele Prisión, Adolfo Garijo, was also the director of the documentary. As Álvaro González writes, the channel had a range of programming for its prison audience, and it 'retransmitía la música que tocaban los presos, los partidos de fútbol y baloncesto que jugaban en el patio. Había una televisión en cada galería para que lo vieran' [it broadcast the music played by the prisoners and the football and basketball games played in the courtyard. There was a television in each cellblock for them to watch] (González 2020). As reporters were unlikely to venture into Carabanchel, 'empezaron a tomar prestadas imágenes y testimonios de Tele Prisión, por lo que la iniciativa empezó a conocerse y tener repercusión en el exterior las demandas y reivindicaciones de los internos' [they began to borrow images and testimonies from Tele Prisión, so the initiative began to be known and the demands and claims of the inmates had an impact on the outside] (González 2020). Its success in Carabanchel was short-lived, however. When the documentary was financed and distributed by Radio Televisión Madrid (Tele Madrid) in 1987, its public projection and distribution prompted the near-immediate cessation of the Tele Prisión project (and reprisals for the prisoners who directed and participated in it). Given the images documented in the film, it is not difficult to imagine what provoked such swift retribution.

The documentary opens with light, jaunty music and images of sunshine and green grass—a park or open space where two people walk on a path together. Gradually, darker and deeper chords penetrate this music as the camera cuts to aerial shots of Carabanchel's spoked panopticon. The camera cuts again to a row of trees over a hilly, bucolic vista, the jaunty music dominating the moody chords that had interrupted it. Zooming slowly out, the audience sees more of the surrounding environment and the camera reveals an open patio surrounded by a redbrick building, which eventually reveals that this scene is being filmed from behind bars. The shrill introduction of an organ into the music wails as the title of the documentary flashes across the screen, eventually converting into a high-pitched alarm as prisoners are brought into the Carabanchel complex. The introduction to the documentary thus sharply juxtaposes the lightness and promise of freedom with a weighted, discordant sense of being trapped. Images of lush green fade to red brick, and the curated spryness of the music is interrupted by darker and more sinister chords that speak to the violence of being imprisoned. The voiceover to the documentary describes the prison in similarly dark ways, speaking over these images: 'Carabanchel: una ciudad dentro de la ciudad. Un pozo. Uno se pregunta "¿Qué seres viven entre estos hierros, entre estas rejas y cerrojos?"' [Carabanchel: a city within the city. A cesspool. One wonders 'What beings live between these iron bars, between these bars and padlocks?'] (Garijo 1987).

It is a mistake to say that the documentary is merely critical of the conditions of Carabanchel, as these conditions are wholly apparent from the outset. Simply filming the galleries and cells demonstrates the poor hygiene, filth, and infestations with which these prisoners lived. The voiceover notes the facts of Carabanchel, describing how the prison

> fue concebida para unos 900 internos, y alberga en la actualidad una cifra que oscila entre los 2300 y los 2500. Prácticamente todos son presos preventivos; es decir, que no han sido juzgados todavía. Según el ordenamiento jurídico español, pueden permanecer en prisión hasta cuatro años en la espera de juicio. (Garijo 1987)[9]

As noted before, the peculiarity of the Spanish penal system meant that someone who had committed a minor infraction could be subject to the same fatal conditions as an inmate condemned to life in prison. Minutes

9 '[I]t was conceived for some 900 inmates, and currently houses a number that ranges between 2,300 and 2,500. Virtually all of them are remand prisoners; that is, they have not yet been tried. According to the Spanish legal system, they can remain in prison for up to four years while awaiting trial.'

later, a prisoner puts this even more succinctly: 'Aquí estamos condenados por condena de muerte por el asunto de la enfermedad del SIDA' [We're sentenced to death here because of AIDS] (Garijo 1987).

It is clear to see how an inmate might feel this way, amid the sick and dying. The rampant infection rates in Spain likely only served to increase the pervading sense of being surrounded by AIDS. As Arroyo-Cobo writes: 'By the end of the 1980s, the HIV infection rate in injecting drug users in the community was nearly 60%. The number of this type of drug user amongst prisoners was almost 50% so it was therefore understandable that infection rates in prisons were about 30%' (2010, 630). Though the Fundamental General Prison Act of 1979 standardized 'medical assistance in penitentiary settings as a responsibility of the Prison Administration' (Arroyo-Cobo 2010, 630), a notable reform over the human rights violations of the Francoist dictatorship, the shunting of responsibility to the Prison Administration forced inmates to rely on an institutional definition of wellbeing and healthcare. In the case of Carabanchel, dependence on the generosity and care of the administration kept prisoners sick, unwashed, and in dangerous conditions.

The inmates in *Carabanchel: la otra orilla* unanimously protest these conditions. One says that 'no tenemos ni agua, el servició está roto, si sale el agua por abajo, y aquí el estado da 280 pesetas por cada preso y no nos dan ni 20 duros de comida...' [we don't even have water, the toilet is broken and toilet water comes out from underneath it, and here the state gives 280 pesetas for each prisoner and they don't even give us 100 pesetas for food], while another declares that 'hay mucha suciedad. ¿Cómo no vamos a tener SIDA, cómo no vamos a tener sífilis y ... enfermedades, si la base de todo es que no hay higiene? No hay higiene, no se reparte lejía en suficientes cantidades ... [o] jabón ... Se nos dan los rollos de papel higiénico al mes' [there is a lot of filth. How could we not get AIDS, how could we not get syphilis and ... diseases, if the basis of everything is that there is no hygiene? There is no hygiene, and bleach is not distributed in sufficient quantities ... [or] soap ... We [only] get toilet paper rolls monthly] (Garijo 1987). Alongside their statements, the camera continues to display shots of chipped paint on the walls through the bars of individual cells, dirty sinks, water-stained walls and floors, mold and mildew darkening nearly every crevice. A prisoner urinates into a toilet, the corner where he is standing discolored and yellowed.

While the hygienic conditions in the prison keep the prisoners sick, visits to the doctor are strictly rationed. The documentary describes the process of requesting a medical appointment, which occurs on one day, with the actual visit taking place the next day, after which the inmate may receive medicine on the third day. As the documentary shows, the lack of prompt attention drives some inmates to self-harm while others look to escape through sex or drugs. The same sorts of risky activities that create spikes of infection in the general population undergird the desperate search for sensation in prison; needles, in particular, are frequently shared for tattoos and drug use. One prisoner, speaking of common drug practices in Carabanchel, says that 'para darte un pico tienes que coger una jeringa de la basura y pincharte con ella, o afilar la aguja, o darle mantequilla ... O sea, cosas de esas, y con la misma chuta pues nos podemos picar 20 personas' [to shoot up you have to take a syringe from the garbage and use it, or [you have to] sharpen the needle, or add heroin ... I mean, things like that, and with the same junk, 20 people could shoot up] (Garijo 1987). Needle-exchange programs, which would eventually reduce the cross-infection of needle sharing in spaces like Carabanchel, were not established in Spain until 1997.[10] In the meantime, the type of practices described by this prisoner would continue to produce outbreaks and multiple infections.

Carabanchel: la otra orilla frames the prisoners of Carabanchel not as individuals but as an oppressed collective: they are not named, are sometimes anonymized as voices or shadowed figures, and voice near-unanimous concerns about the prison. The similarities of their stories blend together, a chorus which often—and rightly so—laments the treatment and conditions of Carabanchel as infernal. They exhort the viewer, calling for compassion and advocating for fair and humane treatment or simple acknowledgment of the conditions in the prison. Hearing their stories recalls the ghosted ruins that Edensor describes, those overladen spaces that still thrum with an excess of memory. I do not argue that these prisoners should be seen as ghosts, and in so doing that we should detachedly regard their pleas as fiction, story, or ethereal and unimportant; instead, I see the documentary as showing how 'haunting is not thus merely a psychological projection but is imbricated in the relationships between people and places, and this

10 In 1985 the government took formal control of methadone administration, and its use was eventually approved for prisons (see Real Decreto 75/1990). Other harm-reduction programs, such as community-run needle-exchange programs, had also been in place in Spain since 1988 in Barcelona and Bilbao (Romero Vallecillos et al. 2005, 260). This was not the case in Spanish prisons, however, which were much slower to adopt needle-exchange programs. Following a 1995 initiative in the Basque Country that encouraged the creation of a pilot needle-exchange program, the prison of Basauri in Bizkaia ran a successful pilot program from 1997 to 1999 that eventually paved the way for other similar programs across Spain. For more information on the methodology, format, and results of the Basauri needle-exchange program, see Aguirre Esunza et al. (n.d.).

includes the material excess, the affordances of ruins, and the performances which are required to negotiate them' (Edensor 2005, 837). The relationship between these prisoners and Carabanchel haunts the reality and legacy of the prison itself, tainting and shaping the simplified ways that HIV/AIDS have been understood in Spain.

As we have seen, the documentary is rife with haunted and haunting moments. The people we see onscreen are angry and resigned, manic and depressed, and occasionally joyful and laughing. They are also, universally, cracking under the pressure of a system whose primary function is not to offer care and wellbeing. One such haunted figure narrates her situation with increasing pain and desperation. She appears after a sequence showing two transgender inmates frolicking in a shower together, set to airy music and no doubt meant to titillate the viewer, and her appearance is meant to shock in contrast to the bathing beauties. In response, the voiceover intones 'la cara y la cruz de la moneda' [the other side of the coin] (Garijo 1987), positioning this transgender prisoner as the inverse of the two women. Lying on a broken bed, the camera angled up toward her face, she pleads with the audience: 'Yo estoy enferma del SIDA. Que me lleven a un ... a un tratamiento ... o a un especialista, o yo qué sé. Necesito salir de aquí. ¿Cuánto puedo pagar? ... Tres meses' [I am sick with AIDS. They need to take me to a ... to treatment ... or to a specialist, or I don't know. I need to get out of here. How much can I pay? ... Three months.] Her words are jumbled as she begs to be released or transferred and treated for her sickness. She pants while she speaks, short and sharp breaths coming in and out quickly. 'Es que me han dicho cuatro años. Yo llevo dos meses' [It's just that they told me four years. I've been here two months.] Her breathing becomes louder, and she whimpers; the sound of her quick, short breaths overtakes all other sound, a rhythmic and pained soundtrack. The camera zooms out, showing her awkwardly posed on the broken bed. She turns over on it and curls up under a blanket before begging again to be set free.

This woman is ruined. She is hollowed out, shelled by the prison system and by illness. Perhaps even more cruelly, she is also expendable—not only for the prison system but for society at large, which cannot fathom a use, need, or recuperative future for her. It is bleak, this portrait of a life left without choice, and differs from other images and representations seen throughout this book in its bleakness. This is to say that the drug addict and the prisoner living with AIDS (emphatically not always the same person, though we have seen just how frequently linked they were) were not envisioned as avatars of innocence and futurity like the hemophiliac child, nor were they seen simply as self-harming deviants, as was the case with homosexuals; instead, they were presented as dangers to society whose disregard for health and wellbeing represented fundamental and existential threats to theoretically normative ways of being. These types of beliefs also allowed the narrator of 'SIDA: Crece la alarma', an episode of the news program *El Dominical*, to point to the tireless work of clinical physicians while noting that 'mientras se investiga, los heroinómanos, acostumbrados a convivir con la muerte, desprecian el riesgo ante la urgencia del caballo' [while it is being investigated, heroin addicts, accustomed to living with death, ignore the risk in the face of the urgency of smack] (1985). By dehumanizing them as already too close to death, drug users are only ever made dangerous scapegoats in the saga of who is to blame for AIDS.

Afterlives

By 1998, Carabanchel was considered obsolete and was subsequently shuttered. The remaining 2,000 men and 500 women were sent to newer prisons around Madrid. The prison itself was left abandoned, as González-Ruibal and Ortiz write, with 'everything left behind' (2015, 21). So much material remained, in fact, that it was able to be repurposed into an art exhibition in Madrid's Centro de Arte Moderno in April 2010. Titled *Carabanchel, la memoria en ruinas*, the exhibition 'showed a diversity of materials collected after the abandonment. These included documents of the inmates, the prison officers and the authorities: psychosocial reports, inmates' petitions, ordinances, minutes, certificates of entrance and departure, personal letters, and medical prescriptions, among other items' (González-Ruibal and Ortiz 2015, 21). This kind of poaching and scavenging of the bones of Carabanchel would happen over the next decade and throughout the 1990s, and the former prison would sink further into disrepair even as parts of it were repurposed into various other uses:

> desde refugio de familias sin techo, a lugar de peregrinación de los grafiteros de toda España, escenario de prácticas de tiro de la policía y, finalmente, mina de materiales metálicos reutilizables, de la cual durante años cuadrillas de trabajadores clandestinos fueron extrayendo sus innumerables rejas y cerramientos metálicos. (Ortiz García and Martínez Zauner 2016, 6–7)[11]

These aspects of Carabanchel's 'post-prison' existence are never fully

11 '[F]rom a shelter for homeless families, to a pilgrimage site for graffiti artists from all over Spain, a police shooting range and, finally, a mine of reusable metal materials, from which for years groups of clandestine workers would extract its innumerable bars and metal locks.'

removed from the realities of the prison that once stood there. Dominique Moran writes that 'whatever the purpose (if any) to which a prison site is subsequently put, vestiges of its previous function remain inscribed in its cultural landscape, whether these are uncomfortable reminders, commercially attractive qualities, or a combination of the two' (2015, 132). We see this in the artifacts left behind in the ruins of Carabanchel, the dilapidated and crumbling buildings themselves, and also in its afterlives, as the prison was torn down and repurposed. In 2008, and despite protests advocating that the site be converted into a national historic monument or preserved in some way under the Law of Historical Memory, the primary building of Carabanchel was demolished. Ortiz García and Zauner describe post-prison Carabanchel thus:

> La desaparición del edificio convirtió una construcción que durante diez años fue una ruina, evocadora de su existencia como lugar de represión, en un ámbito vacío donde algunos grupos todavía hoy se empeñan en convocar, como si de un espectro se tratara, el espíritu de los que allí sufrieron prisión por motivo de su ideología, su orientación sexual o su lucha sindical; en suma por la defensa de las libertades. (Ortiz García and Martínez Zauner 2016, 12)[12]

Following Moran, it seems telling that this space, built on the backs of prisoners and maintained in a deplorable condition for decades, was unable to be fully rehabilitated. The ephemeral spaces that emerged and vanished in its decade of crumbling toward demolition speak to the long history of state oppression and state-sanctioned violence that the prison represents. Groups like *Plataforma por un centro para la paz y la memoria en la antigua cárcel de Carabanchel* have decried the razing of the building and continue to advocate for a museum of historical memory to replace it, while other neighborhood associations argue for livable spaces like grocery stores, residences, and community areas. Instead, in June of 2005, an immigrant detention center ('Centro de internamiento de extranjeros', or CIE) was opened in what was formerly Carabanchel's prison hospital. Rather than referencing the deep history and infamy of the site, the center is most commonly referred to as the 'CIE in Madrid' or, perhaps only slightly

12 'The disappearance of the building transformed a structure that for ten years had been a ruin, evocative of its existence as a place of repression, into an empty space where some groups still strive today to summon, as if it were a specter, the spirit of the those who were imprisoned there for their ideological beliefs, their sexual orientation or their fight for labor conditions; in short, for the defense of freedoms.'

more infrequently, as the 'CIE in Aluche', one of the neighborhoods that border the detention center. The metaphorical relocation of the site from Carabanchel to Aluche (or even more broadly, a nebulous description of a location somewhere in Madrid) works to hide the prison by covering up its past and its notoriety, an attempt to whitewash its façade. Notwithstanding these attempts to scrub Carabanchel clean, the failure to imagine anything beyond a new 'detention center'—itself a euphemistic turn that seeks to avoid the imagery of the prison—is a measure of Carabanchel's imprint on the cultural and geographical memory.

While the prison's central building and galleries were being demolished in 2008, the local government of Madrid promised the construction of mixed-use housing, retail areas, and a hospital. As of 2022, the space sits empty still, a field that is slowly creeping over the bricks and detritus left behind. The history of this site—not only because of its ties to the fascist dictatorship of Francisco Franco, but in its human rights abuses and health violations—seems sown into the ground. For this reason, perhaps the absence of a promised hospital is itself an echo of Carabanchel's legacy as a site that saw HIV/AIDS proliferate, an irony too great for the physical space to withstand. In a parallel fashion, the inability of the former hospital to contain or even empathetically care for people with AIDS becomes further underscored in its conversion to a detention center. In short, we see here a prison hospital that can only serve as prison, and an empty space that cannot be imagined as anything other than haunted by the memory of the prison.

In this way, perhaps Carabanchel and Escuelas Pías are exemplary ruins of HIV/AIDS. By this I mean that the ruins created alongside and by AIDS are seen at once to be eyesores but erasable, objects to be bulldozed out of the narrative or physically razed. Of course, the same applies for people with AIDS: whether through the deliberate selection of a 'perfect victim' by the media, the solidification of communities as sexual predators, or the incarceration of hapless reprobates, people with AIDS were codified and made to fit a crafted narrative of who falls outside the borders of the community and state. In the Escuelas Pías, there is no trace of the drug users or people with HIV who once inhabited its crumbling walls. Instead, we have a modernized architectural work that leaps backward in time to the origins of the site, papering over the cracks in its storied history. With Carabanchel, the site itself eventually crumbled into obsolence, housing groups of Roma, itinerants, graffiti artists, and scavengers before finally being razed. The remaining building, once the prison hospital, became an immigrant detention center, and state-sanctioned violence is thus reified, including and especially through a site long seen as emblematic of such violence.

The eminently erasable addict cannot be reformed, but must be removed from the narrative. When I speak of the stories created from feeling sick, there is an imprint of a person here, or an excavated cavity—in short, a lack—where people who used drugs might once have had a voice regarding their suffering, treatment, and care while living with HIV. Samuel Amago has written that

> the State ensures that discards disappear from our lived environments, but trash never vanishes. Our contact with things represents only a fraction of the long life of those things, since after they have been ejected from the realm of human use, discards keep on existing, exerting their vital material force in ways that are not always visible: leaking, leaching, decaying, evaporating, decomposing, remaining. (2019, 146–47)

We may think of places—Escuelas Pías, Carabanchel Prison—in this manner. We may also think the same of people; not in a way that furthers the injustices and inequalities they have been subjected to, but instead in a manner that honors and recounts their experience as important, worth remembering, and unjustly lived. The truth of the matter is that for drug users, their narrative was written by others, perhaps more forcefully and more powerfully so than we have seen in previous chapters. The moments where the stories of their illnesses and treatment break through, as we have seen in *Carabanchel: la otra orilla*, reveal the extent of their erasure from the national story of HIV/AIDS. They live on in flashing images, forgotten and demolished spaces, in memory, and as discards that continue to move, pressure, and remain with us.

Conclusion:

The Plague of the Twentieth Century

AIDS has been called many things since it was first diagnosed, and many of its names and epithets have been recounted in these pages: red plague, gay plague, gay cancer, gay-related immune deficiency, and the plague of the twentieth century, to name just a few. The perceptions and feelings toward it have mutated and evolved as time passes; not necessarily in a traceable, progressive manner, but in fits and starts. Understanding HIV/AIDS, for that reason, is perhaps best seen as a process that touches nerve centers and electrifies social and cultural fears of contagion, illness, queerness, blood, and more.

This was not understood in the early 1980s, as this book has made apparent. Instead, epidemiological institutions traced incomplete outbreak narratives, which in turn delineated contagious culprits and their victims; national governments dismissed dangers, ignored risks, and blamed socially marginalized groups for the increasing spread of AIDS; and televised news and print media came up with a cast of bad actors and crafted new and sensational epidemiological narratives for their confused and poorly informed readership. This is the macro-narrative of the epidemic in its early years—the broad history of the pandemic, as much as it can be pieced together and as we have seen in each chapter of this book. The micro-stories of HIV/AIDS—those individualized and personal stories of living through, with, or in spite of the illness—tell different tales of what AIDS was like in these early years. Sometimes these stories intersect, as in the journalism of Jordi Petit (2003), who places the crisis of representation under which the LGBTQ community suffered in Spain in critical dialog with medical and cultural institutions at the time. Other times these stories seem almost nonsensical, ill-fitting, or at odds with larger narratives, as could be the case with 'S.I.D.A' by Peor Impossible, 'SIDA da' by Las Pekinesas, or in the ephemera produced by groups like the Movimiento de Liberación Gay de Euskal Herria. The outbreak narrative is the macro-story, the purported truth of the matter as told by authorities and institutions; the micro-story is your perspective, or that of your neighbor, cousin, or friend, and tells your story of survival through an ongoing crisis.[1]

In each chapter, I have worked to document and demonstrate the effect of living through history in the making, and the effect that this has on one's ability to articulate the experience of living through a crisis. It can be messy business, and it sometimes doesn't make sense. Why was there not greater public outrage in Spain regarding the developing government control over marginal communities, control which emerged amid a heady upswelling of support for democracy during the Transition? Or how does one reconcile the fact that one's own experience of living through the initial HIV/AIDS crisis does not match up to the narratives of silence, ignorance, or criminal neglect seen here? In part, this is because the history of the event has been written by institutional forces and structures. The same institutions that struggled to care for the lives of Spanish citizens have been able to write the post-outbreak narrative: uncertainties become fixed truths, lives are erased, and injustices are bulldozed over. Inching closer to the lived experience of the epidemic—the micro-histories that are, of course, never singular, never fixed, and always partial—has been one of this book's main goals.

A structure of feeling sick, as we have seen throughout this book, is multivocal, equivocating, and cacophonous. It returns to Raymond Williams's original formation of a structure of feeling, which Diedrich synthesizes by noting Williams's desire to 'think about how cultural productions ... capture forming and formative processes without making them into formed wholes' (Diedrich 2016, 48). That is to say that, when living through history-in-the-making, multiple explosive events are happening at the same time, creating meanings of differing scale and importance to a developing macro-history; because of this, it is possible to have a gay man presenting AIDS-related illnesses after travel, two hemophiliac children in Sevilla living in poverty and receiving posthumous media attention, and a forgotten drug user in Barcelona who sometimes slept with men, all living and dying nearly concurrently but with vastly different experiences, ramifications, and visibility. It is further possible to have prison riots and incendiary footage about HIV in Carabanchel, or LGBTQ groups holding demonstrations, parades, and activist actions, and still find panels of medical experts and political actors cracking jokes and dithering over the importance of AIDS to the public at large. Seeing the plurality of voices in

1 I am indebted to Julián Daniel Gutiérrez-Albilla for the gentle probing that has allowed me to articulate the distinctions between the macro- and micro-histories of HIV/AIDS in these early years.

a structure of feeling sick is to recognize the social affect of the times as a kaleidoscopic mass of rage, hope, joy, loss, death, and life.

Blood and monsters

This book has focused on the earliest years of AIDS in Spain (1981–1986) precisely because the sense of history-in-formation is so profound during this period. By 1987, there was both a test for HIV antibodies and early therapeutic approval for the drug azidothymidine, or AZT, both of which would change the narratives surrounding HIV/AIDS dramatically. The pre-treatment era, marked as it was by uncertainty, was thus distinct from a subsequent era in which substantive medical intervention was finally possible.[2] Up to that point, and by 1986, Spain's numbers of people with AIDS had jumped dramatically from its first cases, thoroughly disproving the myth that the illness could remain relegated to the foreign shores of the United States or within a select group of marginal communities. In news reports and TV specials, however, AIDS remained a niche illness in many ways, an epidemic primarily associated with the same risk groups to which it had been attached since the earliest days of the epidemic. The media accounts of this time, then, colored the experience of the epidemic in a way that was crucial to its broad perception. While AIDS may have been experienced in ways that were at once multiple, complex, and rich during this period, representations of the illness funneled it into a bleak message of terror and death. To name a particularly salient example, when the AIDS drama *An Early Frost* (John Erman, 1985) made its television debut in the United States, it was the first fictionalized cinematic account of the illness. In Spain, the national television channel RTVE translated the title as *Diagnóstico Fatal: SIDA* [*Fatal Diagnosis: AIDS*]. The Spanish title cut to the bone of the matter, summarizing the sourness of illness into a single, obvious outcome: death. As we have seen time and again, the linkages established in this moment and across other televised media from Spain cemented the story of AIDS as horrific and threatening, the terrifying result of hedonistic practices and willfully villainous seeders of the virus.

If the proliferating epithets for HIV/AIDS were so common in these early years, it is at least in part because AIDS was always considered monstrous.

2 It should be noted that early treatments with AZT were effective, in a broad sense, though they came with significant side-effects in the doses they were initially administered. For more about the dilemma of AZT use, see Garfield's article in *The Independent* (2011). In a more thorough account of the history of HIV/AIDS-related therapies, Samuel Broder (2010) details the approval times, clinical trials, and treatment dates for the drugs that would come to be used to treat HIV/AIDS.

Such monstrosity existed not just because of the illness's mysterious origins, but because of its debilitating physical effects, fatality, and virulence. AIDS appeared to be everywhere at once, culling friends and families with abandon, and seemingly unstoppable. There were, subsequently, a range of feelings about the threat of HIV/AIDS that gave way to any number of attempts to mitigate anxiety, cope with loss, laugh away the threat, or ignore its potential. I have indicated throughout this book that some of these attempts to describe HIV/AIDS at this time could be seen as 'bad' products in the way that they ran counterproductive to progressive activism and attempts to curb the increasingly desperate fear toward the perceived risk groups of AIDS. A structure of feeling sick isn't always productive, nor does it always get things right; it is an expression of one's relationship to the present, an attempt to feel one's way forward in time. The richness of such expressions has its own importance, though, and understanding how we felt around so blindly in the past can offer a way forward through the present.

In the remainder of this conclusion, I turn to something that may be considered a 'bad' product, in no small part because its author was always so keen on capitalizing on bad affects. In what seems to have been an attempt to harness the fear of HIV/AIDS as well as the silence surrounding its cinematic representation, Jesús 'Jess' Franco—one of Spain's most prolific and mythologized B-movie directors—wrote and directed the first 'AIDS film' to be made in Spain in 1986, *SIDA: La peste del siglo XX* [*AIDS: The Plague of the Twentieth Century*]. Franco's film never saw the light of day, however, due to strong disagreements between the director and the production company (a not uncommon occurrence for the outspoken Franco).[3] The film captures the mystery and terror surrounding AIDS in 1986 in sensational ways—particularly by portraying the virus as a malevolent, androgynous alien force bent on sexually conquering the world. Franco's fantastic vision of the illness wrapped up fatal sexuality, mysterious transmission methods, and fears of queerness in a frenetic package.

AIDS: The Plague of the Twentieth Century opens on a young man, Matt, beating on a door and screaming the name of his lover, Danny. An old woman answers the door, and after a brief exchange with her, Matt learns that Danny has been locked in his room for days. Matt enters the apartment and, at the door to Danny's room, pleads to be let in. Behind the door, Danny is stoic

3 The result of the disagreement left the film unedited as well as undistributed. At least one copy of the film's negatives currently languishes in the Madrid Film Archives, where it is unable to be screened. The script of the film, as well as a handful of photographs taken during filming, are available in the National Library of Spain in Madrid. This chapter's analysis is based on the film's script and character cues.

and resolved, refusing Matt entry and insisting that he leave. From their conversation through the door, the audience learns that Danny has ended the relationship rather mysteriously and that Matt has become desperate to understand why. Finally convincing Danny to open the door, Matt exclaims '¡Dios mío!' [My God!] upon seeing him, to which Danny replies '¿Comprendes ahora por qué no quería verte?' [Do you understand now why I didn't want to see you?] Matt's only reply to Danny's pained question is the brief 'es atroz' [it's awful]. 'Sí', Danny says, 'Tengo el sida' [I have AIDS] (Franco 1986). Based on its screenplay directions, this conversation appears to have been filmed with Danny's face and expression off-camera until the momentous reveal of his disfigurement through illness. As the scene continues, Danny explains: 'Fui a ver a un doctor. Me dijo que no podia hacer nada por mí. Llevo el virus en la sangre' [I went to see a doctor. He told me there was nothing he could do for me. I carry the virus in my blood.] The camera cuts again to Danny, who admits: 'Voy a morir' [I'm going to die.] The camera here serves as both judge and jury for Danny, looking away from him until crucial moments that both reveal and revel in the visibility of his affliction. As the script notes show, Franco utilizes voiceover between the two lovers for most of this sequence. Danny is shown hidden behind a door or with his back to the camera, for example, underscoring the mysteriousness of whatever is ailing him. His admission of AIDS is the first moment that he appears on camera, after which the script returns to voiceovers until he confesses that he is going to die. Franco plays a quick game of hide-and-seek here, tantalizing the viewer with horror and only revealing it in sharp melodramatic shocks. At the same time, he offers an unsubtle linkage between AIDS and death—one that is based not only on its grotesque physicality, as he imagines it, but on the belief in its inevitability. Of course, Franco was only taking his cues from the types of scandalized news media that I have examined throughout this book, which so often showed people with AIDS as debilitated and riddled with the telltale purple lesions of Kaposi's sarcoma. As the camera cuts away from Danny's pronouncement of his own death, Matt pleadingly cries, '¿Por qué te fuiste con él, Danny, teniéndome a mí? ¡Puede que me hayas contagiado también!' [Why did you go with him, Danny, when you had me? You could have infected me as well!] Through voiceover, Danny abruptly says goodbye to Matt and, although the screenplay is sparse here, he appears to jump out of a window to his death.

This melodramatic establishing sequence of what the virus is, what it is capable of, and how it kills is, clearly, a highly sensationalized account of HIV/AIDS, even by the loose standards of representation in 1986. Nevertheless, the heightened account of AIDS found here in many ways follows the journalistic precedent established by contemporary media reports of the period in Spain and elsewhere, as recounted in Chapter 1. This is to say that *AIDS: The Plague of the Twentieth Century* tells a gruesome story of hideously afflicted lovers doomed to death and suicide, but it was hardly alone in doing so.[4] In a very real way, then, Franco's film follows the discourse of the time, as Spaniards were watching weekly reports whose titles breathlessly oscillated between complacency and wholesale panic: 'Alarm: The Virus that Comes from California' (1983); 'AIDS: The Illness of the 80s' (1983); 'AIDS: The Enigma can be Solved' (1984); 'AIDS in San Francisco: Panic in the Streets' (1985); 'AIDS: The Growing Alarm' (1985); 'AIDS in Spain: The Syndrome of the Syndrome' (1986); 'Homosexuals: The Crisis of AIDS' (1987), to name but a handful. The brief opening vignette of Franco's doomed lovers thus borrows from a variety of sources in order to structure its narrative: not only the tears and panic of the melodramatic 'weepie' or the creeping tension between the seen and the unseen often found in the horror genre, but the sensationalized journalistic spectacle of the body in pain. In capturing the 'bodily excess' of the filmic genres of horror and melodrama, Franco offers up what Linda Williams has called the 'spectacle of a body caught in the grip of intense sensation or emotion' (1991, 4), while also providing a singular thrill for an audience who, ostensibly, would never experience the very real devastation of AIDS. The result is a fantastic film that is wrapped up in melodramatic excess, fear, and almost pornographic sensationalism.[5]

The remainder of *AIDS: The Plague of the Twentieth Century* retools a semblance of medical fact with urban myth and conspiracy theory, positing the virus as a sexually transmitted threat that is brought about by an androgynous alien species seeking to dominate Earth. Those infected by the alien AIDS supervirus die in mere days, but in the meantime serve as carriers for a weakened virus that can be passed to other humans, which is revealed to be HIV. The alien race seeding it through the populace, known collectively as Andros, tears through heterosexual families visiting tropical locales, homosexual couples, and unsuspecting virgins; the virus's spread is in this manner loosely fenced in along the lines of risk groups,

4 Readers familiar with *An Early Frost* (1985), *Longtime Companion* (1989), or *Philadelphia* (1993) will easily see how the Franco film is hardly exceptional in its portrayal of the AIDS trope of the doomed lover and his visibly marked face and body.

5 This is familiar territory for Franco, whose 150+ films quite often straddled the borders between erotic cinema and terror in a fantastic B-movie aesthetic. For more on Franco's films and legacy, see Balbo and Blumenstock's groundbreaking book on his work, *Obsession: The Films of Jess Franco* (1993) as well as Lázaro-Reboll and Olney's edited volume *The Films of Jess Franco* (2018).

risky practices, and exotic, foreign dens of pleasure. As in real life, people are snatched away quickly, others are left behind to ponder their own vulnerability, and a select few remain behind and warn others about the impending doom.

What is significant about Franco's film is how viscerally it encapsulates the fear and monstrosity in which HIV/AIDS was mired in these early years. Its open embrace of B-movie aesthetics and grotesque sexuality allows it to revel in the types of AIDS narratives that were wildly prevalent at the time, and in so doing it gives voice to a range of emotions, conspiracies, and fears. This is, of course, precisely what might make it a bad object for some. But structures of feeling are not always voiced in popular, progressive, or neutral ways from the outset—sometimes they flail, sometimes they are gross or disturbing, and sometimes they offend. So, in spite of its supernatural and fantastical content (and in some ways, because of it), Franco's film is able to express a particular experience of existing with and around HIV/AIDS at this time—not through a neutral or sympathetic lens, but through one that nevertheless captures the social fears and popular horror of AIDS at the time.

A particularly salient example of this occurs in the immediate aftermath of Danny's suicide. In this sequence, one of the film's main characters, Dr. Hausman, is performing an autopsy on Danny's body. He narrates the results, stating that 'al hacer la autopsia del joven Danny Banks se descubrió que el virus del sida le había atacado con una violencia y una rapidez extrema. Desde años atrás Danny y Matt había sido una pareja inseparable y fiel...' [an autopsy on young Danny Banks revealed that the AIDS virus had attacked him with extreme violence and speed. For years, Danny and Matt had been an inseparable and faithful couple] (Franco 1986). The echoes of the earliest medical article on AIDS in Spain are undeniable. As seen in Chapter 1, that report ran through the patient's symptoms while describing his 'stable, one-partner relationship' and the fact that 'during visits to New York in 1974 and Turkey in 1980 he had had sexual contacts with different partners' and 'repeated episodes of gonorrhea' (Vilaseca et al. 1982, 572). In both texts, stability and fidelity are held aloft as markers of committed relationships so that they may be contrasted with the wanton abandon and hedonism of gay sexuality; and in both texts, AIDS becomes the obvious causal result of straying outside the safe borders of the monogamous couple.

In the film, Dr. Hausman's autopsy voiceover hammers this idea home:

> Una mañana, algunos días antes de que Danny empezara a presentar síntomas visibles del síndrome, la abuela de Danny vio salir de la alcoba

> del muchacho a alguien inesperado, una bellísima dama. Silenciosa, ausente, pasó ante la anciana ignorándola. Y solo a salir se despidió. Su voz era grave, profunda, demasiado profunda para ser la voz de una mujer. (Franco 1986)[6]

The surprise of Danny's surmised tryst with a beautiful woman initially seems to suggest a sort of queerness to his homosexuality, a pansexually lascivious sickness in what was initially portrayed as wholesome, monogamous homosexuality—a winsome couple whose quintessential American names only lend to the perception of their ruby-cheeked goodness. The strangeness of the woman (and the final lines that intimate that this was, in fact, not a woman) further informs the perception of Danny's adultery as particularly odd or sexually aberrant. Portraying Danny's lover as a gravelly-voiced woman toys with a kind of popularly perceived aberration that is at once disgusting, exciting, frightening, titillating, and sexually provocative. The film furthers this narrative when the audience learns that she is Andros, the androgynous alien collective that has been superspreading HIV through the population, which only serves to heighten the perception of her purported strangeness.

This sort of interest in the aberrant body—here, an oversexualized yet alien body that is marked by HIV/AIDS—is nothing new for Franco or his work. Tatjana Pavlović, for example, describes Franco's work as obsessively centering bodies. Because of their centrality, she argues,

> Franco's bodies pose a threat and a question. He demonstrates that there is no natural body that does not involve a social and a cultural dimension; Franco's transgressive bodies upset notions of order and hierarchy. He envisions an alternative social order, unraveling and unsettling the social hierarchy with its clear gender relations. (2003, 118)

This is done through an obsessive heightening of bodies: beautiful but deadly mad scientists, horrifically mutilated corpses, powerful and idealized superheroes, and hypersexual erotic vampires, to name a few of the long list of characters that populate his films. Unlike in his other films, however, Franco does very little to upend the social order here, as

6 'One morning, a few days before Danny began to show visible symptoms of the illness, his grandmother saw someone unexpected come out of the boy's bedroom—a beautiful lady. Silent and distracted, she passed the old woman, ignoring her. And only as she was leaving did she say goodbye. Her voice was low, deep, too deep to be a woman's voice.'

it had already been upended by HIV/AIDS. That is, the addition of alien sex vampires beaming down to give everyone AIDS could almost be read as just another conspiracy theory in a long line of them, another urban myth to add to the ones that were already being heavily propagated at this time.[7] Franco's work here, then, does not create an alternative social order as much as it documents the way that the social order had already been confounded by AIDS. In short, the confusion, disruption, and fear echoing through the film were already in place; Franco just capitalized on it, adding another sort of fantasy to the already fantastical musings and misinformation surrounding the illness.

In ways that are both fascinating and frightening, Franco's work seems ripe for the pandemic landscape of the early 1980s. Writing on Franco's relationship to genre cinema, Tim Lucas classified his filmography as 'horrotica', a genre 'responsible for wedding the thrills of cinematic sex and horror into a third *frisson*' (1993, 13). Lucas goes on to say that 'in Franco's universe, the viewer never encounters joyous sex; there is always some dark element of guilt or pain or emotional dislocation involved, and most of the erotic acts he depicts are dramatized in concert with the specter of Death' (1993, 13). *SIDA: La peste del siglo XX* is no different, and the specter of death and illness looming over sex is seen throughout the film. Soon after the initial sequence of the two lovers, the audience is introduced to Bill Monihan and Dr. Simone Rouquier, who both begin to work with Dr. Hausman in order to study the strange sex-related deaths that are now becoming more and more frequent. Dr. Hausman introduces Bill and Simone to Victor/Miss Linda, a patient of his who is being treated for the cerebral lesions that have (supposedly) scrambled her brain and her perception of her sex. Miss Linda reveals herself to have been ravaged by Andros prior to the events of the film. She wistfully dreams of Andros, explaining to Dr. Hausman in a session that 'es un príncipe ... A veces puede ser diabólico ... A veces parece un dios' [He is a prince ... Sometimes he can be diabolical ... Sometimes he seems like a god] (Franco 1986). This

7 Many readers will be familiar with the types of myths and conspiracies to which I am referring, and which I described briefly in Chapter 2. Origin myths included its creation as a biological weapon of terror in a laboratory, its zoophilic and barbarous cross-species jump, or a fantastical extraterrestrial or vampiric genesis; various urban myths that it engendered were related to accidental needle pricks, villainous HIV-positive superspreaders like Gaetan Dugas, or a commonly told story of a one-night stand after which the partner (often a woman) leaves her hapless date a message scrawled on their mirror: 'Welcome to the world of AIDS.' See Goldstein (2004) for an excellent study of these types of mythic narratives of AIDS.

conflation of Andros as prince, devil, and god—along with the gift of his sex, which is capable of converting Victor into Miss Linda—malevolently twists sex and death together throughout the film.

As the trio begin to piece together what is happening, they are told the strange story of Augusta Island, which is said to be off the coast of Panama. During the celebration of Carnival, the homosexual populations of Augusta and its surrounding islands get together 'en una explosión de exhibicionismo y desenfado que nadie rechaza durante las fiestas. Luego, aquella sociedad tercermundista vuelve a las convenciones más provincianas y los pederastas vuelven a la clandestinidad' [in an explosion of exhibitionism and disinhibition that no one denies during the holidays. Then, that Third World society returns to the most provincial conventions and its queers go underground.] The result of these festivities, it is learned, are 'special' cases of AIDS in which men who were never suspected of homosexuality are suddenly attacked by the virus after a very short period of incubation. Though the emphasis is on the short incubation period (which, in the logic of the film, suggests the malevolent presence of Andros), the punchline of the story marries perversion with sexual pleasure in a way that always produces death. Further, the focus of this story is decidedly on the otherwise heterosexual men who participate in the hedonistic pleasures of this island Carnival, not the homosexuals who would also be suffering from the results of their purported excesses. This story ultimately serves as a brief window into many of the popular theories surrounding AIDS: from its primordial origins (here, an isolated and backward island in the Caribbean) to its focus on the strange suddenness of viral transmission to, finally, its complete erasure of the communities who would most suffer from it. The horror of this story is not that gay people might die, but that straight people would be caught up in—and fall victim to—their perversions.

This scenario is repeated in the film through Bill, one of the film's leads, for heightened effect. Shortly after meeting Miss Linda, Bill is attacked by Andros. Over the next few sequences, he begins to frequent seedy nightclubs of increasingly ill repute, eventually heading to gay bars. Simone and Hausman begin to follow him, confused by his behavior. The audience learns he is looking for Andros, though he is warned off his search by the patrons of the bars he visits. In the last bar, a group of men titter about Bill's relationship to Andros as the alien approaches him. Speaking to Andros, one of the men tells him:

> Hazle sufrir. Estoy seguro que es masoquista, y además es muy tímido. Bueno a lo mejor tú ya te lo has puesto y te estás quedando con nosotros.

> ¿Lo conocías de antes? Di, ¿ya te lo has trincao? ... No le mires tan fijo que lo estás derritiendo, pobrecillo. Es un chaval bastante guapo.[8]

Bill's response is only to utter 'Andros' before the scene goes black. In the following scenes, an increasingly disfigured Bill makes feverish attempts to return to Simone and Hausman, eventually falling too sick to return to them. They find him at the home of a group of gay men, where he explains that he was attempting to help the pair find Andros and put a stop to the continued outbreak, but that he was entranced by Andros and was unable to escape. Bill dies soon after.

The temptations of the Andros collective—who are described as women, men, and non-binary sexpots throughout the film—are unmatched, but speak of a dark fear of androgyny, queerness, and sex. The fears of tainted queerness echo what we saw in Chapter 2, in the discussion of how HIV/AIDS tainted the perceptions of childhood and hemophiliacs in Spain, even as they were seen as the ultimate victims of the epidemic. By appearing to convert hapless men (it is insinuated but unseen that Andros also feeds on women), Andros becomes the specter of AIDS itself; that is, an entity or figure that preys on the purportedly innocent with a mysterious and fatal touch. His precise origins are unknown, he leaves a trail of devastated people in his wake, and he appears unstoppable. He nests in sexually liberal communities, finding a home and destroying everything around him.

It's a heavy metaphor, and one that is at least a little overwrought. HIV at this time was still ravaging communities, but safe sex campaigns like 'Si da, No da' or 'No te piques', both discussed in earlier chapters, were already in place, as were a number of grassroots anti-AIDS community groups throughout Spain. The marriage of death and sex that is present in the film offers one perspective on how the epidemic was seen, but it was not the only one. That is, the fact that sex in Franco's filmography is always darkened with negative affect or death does not take away from its appearance in *SIDA: La peste del siglo XX*. If anything, it clearly shows the popular strains of thought that classified certain types of sex between certain sets of people at this time as inherently risky and perverse. This can coexist—even frictionally, oppositionally—with the knowledge that activists, a variety of community organizers, and even some medical figures were working to combat the ignorance and mystery surrounding HIV/AIDS.

8 'Make him suffer. I'm sure he's a masochist, and he's also very shy. Well maybe you've already screwed him and you're pulling our chains. Did you know him from before? Hey, have you fucked? ... Don't stare at him so hard, you're melting the poor thing. He's a pretty handsome kid.'

By the end of the film, Bill's death has been the last straw for Hausman and Simone, who plan to reveal the truth about AIDS to the world, strange as it may sound. Simone makes a presentation to a group of scientists at an international symposium on AIDS, describing the virus's extraterrestrial origins and the lives that were lost as they made this discovery. In some of the film's final lines, she states:

> Quiero desde aquí rendir homenaje a una de las personas cuyo virus ha sido esencial para nuestras afirmaciones y que ha muerto en mis brazos hace pocos días en aras de la ciencia. Se trate del ayudante ... del Dr. Hausman, Bill Monihan, Dios la [*sic*] bendiga. Podemos afirmar que el virus del SIDA obedece un plan maquiavélico contra la raza humana. (Franco 1986)[9]

In Simone's epitaph on Bill's life, there is a faint echo of the numerous eulogies made in the early years of AIDS, a type of homage to those lost in the middle of an unceasing pandemic. Her strange slip of the tongue, which seems to misgender Bill in the middle of her thoughtful eulogy, seems innocuous until one thinks of how he died—surrounded by a group of gay men after being ravaged and sodomized by Andros. Bill dies as Bill, but even in this slip, something is revealed, perhaps, that shows a vision of Bill as marred: he has been feminized, penetrated by illness, death, and sex.[10] It's a moment not unlike the earlier slippage of the word 'homofílico' [homophiliac], as seen in Chapter 2, another linguistic slip that merged two groups of people into one. Like the apocryphal homophiliac, the typo, error, or misspelling during Bill's eulogy could simultaneously be another moment in which some vision of those with HIV are seen; that is, as a masculinity that bends to something mysterious, deadly, and sexual, and suffers for it.

As Franco's film reminds us, the discourse surrounding the virus was wrapped up in layers of meaning that were at once highly mediated and

9 'Here, I want to pay tribute to one of the people whose virus has been essential to our discoveries and who died in my arms a few days ago for the sake of science: that is, Dr. Hausman's assistant ... Bill Monihan, God bless her [*sic*]. We can affirm that the AIDS virus follows a Machiavellian plan against the human race.'

10 It should be acknowledged that Franco's screenplay is riddled with typos, errors, and edits throughout, and is clearly meant to have been a draft that would have gone unseen beyond a select number of the film's cast and crew. There are grammatical mistakes and frequent misspellings throughout, and sometimes words have been crossed out and replaced. It is thus highly plausible that the error here is unintentional on Franco's part and would have been corrected in filming. As I note above, however, these facts do not diminish the importance of this slippage.

bound to conventions of media genres. The stories told are excessive and designed to provoke audiences, moving them with sensations that might resemble fear or panic, sadness or despair, or morbid sexual titillation. Understanding this confluence, then, becomes crucial for reading the event of the AIDS outbreak not as a story belonging to the past but as one that we still struggle with, not as a singular expressible media event but as an unfolding process of dealing with history as it is being written. I reference the early years of AIDS in this book for a number of reasons, but partly because the stories told in this moment form an amalgamation of a very real horror and excess that was simultaneously unbelievable and almost otherworldly in its destruction.

It seems almost transactional to say that this book is about mining these stories, or that this has been about uncovering them, as if they have not been willfully misplaced, invisibilized, or silenced. Instead, I hope that this book has shown what it means to feel sick, both at this moment and forward in time, as an experience of a sometimes cacophonous, incomplete, and overwhelming mix of narratives that speak to and over each other. It might be unsatisfying at times to know that we cannot fully reveal this past that was so recent, but if anything, it shows how destructive, transformative, and powerful the HIV/AIDS epidemic has been to the social sphere of our lives. Acknowledging the unknowability of feeling sick has allowed this book the space to dismantle some of the originating accounts of the virus, which have served as unstable foundational narratives for something we have yet to fully understand or comprehend; that is, both the illness and virus itself, and the impact and crater-sized hole it has left among us. Ultimately, this book does not reveal some new magic truth about sickness and AIDS, but instead offers something different, an understanding of how we frame illness both literally and figuratively, in the stories we tell and on the screens we watch.

As we move forward—breathing, loving, and interacting with each other—we do so sometimes violently, sometimes unpleasantly, and sometimes uncomfortably. In these connective moments with others, we must see sickness all around us, whether we want to or not, and even as every breath, touch, or kiss blossoms the viral life all around us. It is something we live with and die from. The stories of the early years of AIDS in Spain offer dawning revelations of the deadliness and pleasure of our interactions with each other and our environments. By placing these alongside each other, weaving them together, we are afforded a sense of our place in the interrupting chronologies of illness. In short: a story of feeling sick.

Bibliography

Acevedo, Carlos, ed. 2012. *CT, o, la cultura de la Transición: crítica a 35 años de cultura española*. Actualidad/DeBolsillo 311. Barcelona: DeBolsillo.

Aguirre Esunza, J.A., J.A. Badiola Santamaria, F. Barceló, M. Burón Bengoetxea, M.J. Conde Zabala, V. Fernández de Larrinoa Palacios, K. Gabantxo Laka, et al. n.d. 'El Programa de Intercambio de Jeringuillas de la prisión de Basauri (Bizkaia) (1997–99).' *Ministerio de Sanidad, Servicios Sociales e Igualdad* (blog). https://www.mscbs.gob.es/ciudadanos/enfLesiones/enfTransmisibles/sida/prevencion/progInterJeringuillas/PIJPrisiones/pijEvaluacion.htm. Accessed January 25, 2021.

'Alarma: El virus que viene de California.' 1983. *Informe Semanal*. Madrid: RTVE.

Alcaide, Jesús. 2020. 'Sujeto brillante desidentificado: una lectura entre Miguel Benlloch y José Esteban Muñoz.' In La Madraza: Centro de Cultura Contemporánea. https://lamadraza.ugr.es/multimedia/conferencia-sujeto-brillante-desidentificado-una-lectura-cruzada-entre-miguel-benlloch-y-jose-esteban-munoz/. Accessed October 3, 2022.

Aliaga, Juan Vicente, and José Miguel G. Cortés. 1997. *Identidad y diferencia: sobre la cultura gay en España*. Barcelona: Editorial Gay y Lesbiana.

Amago, Samuel. 2019. 'Waste and Space in Contemporary Spain: Photographic Archaeologies of the Anthropocene.' *Arizona Journal of Hispanic Cultural Studies* 23 (1): 145–66. https://doi.org/10.1353/hcs.2019.0003.

——. 2021. *Basura: Cultures of Waste in Contemporary Spain*. Charlottesville: University of Virginia Press.

Araneta, Aitzole, and Sandra Fernández Garrido. 2016. 'Transfeminist Genealogies in Spain.' Trans. Michael Brasher. *TSQ: Transgender Studies Quarterly* 3 (1–2): 35–39. https://doi.org/10.1215/23289252-3334163.

Arriola, Aimar, and Nancy Garín. 2014. 'Ficciones globales, luchas locales (o distribución de tres documentos de un contra-archivo del sida en construcción).' *L'internationale* (blog). September 4, 2014. http://www.internationaleonline.org/research/politics_of_life_and_death/7_ficciones_globales_luchas_locales_o_distribucion_de_tres_documentos_de_un_contra_archivo_del_sida_en_construccion. Accessed October 3, 2022.

Arroyo-Cobo, J.M. 2010. 'Public Health Gains from Health in Prisons in Spain.' *Public Health* 124 (11): 629–31. https://doi.org/10.1016/j.puhe.2010.08.007.

Asociación Ciudadana Anti-SIDA de Málaga. n.d. *Lesbianas y SIDA*. Flyer.

Auerbach, David M., William W. Darrow, Harold W. Jaffe, and James W. Curran. 1984. 'Cluster of Cases of the Acquired Immune Deficiency Syndrome.' *The American Journal of Medicine* 76 (3): 487–92. https://doi.org/10.1016/0002-9343(84)90668-5.

Baby, Sophie. 2018. *El mito de la Transición pacífica: violencia y política en España (1975–1982)*. Trans. Tomás Fernández Aúz and Beatriz Eguibar. Madrid: Ediciones Akal.

Balbo, Lucas, and Peter Blumenstock, eds. 1993. *Obsession: The Films of Jess Franco*. Berlin: Graf Haufen & Frank Trebbin.

Benlloch, Miguel, Tomás Navarro, and Rafael Villegas. 1984. *SIDA da*. Performance.

Berlant, Lauren. 2011. *Cruel Optimism*. Durham, NC: Duke University Press.

Bogdanich, Walt, and Eric Koli. 2003. '2 Paths of Bayer Drug in 80's: Riskier One Steered Overseas.' *New York Times*, May 22, 2003. http://www.nytimes.com/2003/05/22/business/2-paths-of-bayer-drug-in-80-s-riskier-one-steered-overseas.html. Accessed October 3, 2022.

Bordowitz, Gregg. 2006. *The AIDS Crisis is Ridiculous and Other Writings, 1986–2003*. Ed. James Meyer. Cambridge, MA: MIT Press.

Broder, Samuel. 2010. 'The Development of Antiretroviral Therapy and Its Impact on the HIV-1/AIDS Pandemic.' *Antiviral Research* 85 (1): 1–18. https://doi.org/10.1016/j.antiviral.2009.10.002.

Butler, Judith. 2004. *Gender Trouble*. New York: Routledge.

Butler, Judith, and Paul Rabinow. 2001. 'Dialogue: Antigone, Speech, Performance, Power.' In *Talk, Talk, Talk: The Cultural Life of Everyday Conversation*. Ed. S.I. Salamensky, 37–48. New York: Routledge.

Byrne, Katherine. 2011. *Tuberculosis and the Victorian Literary Imagination*. Cambridge Studies in Nineteenth-Century Literature and Culture 74. Cambridge: Cambridge University Press.

Calonico, Scott, dir. 2015. *When AIDS Was Funny*. https://video.vanityfair.com/watch/the-reagan-administration-s-chilling-response-to-the-aids-crisis. Accessed October 3, 2022.

Campos Marín, Ricardo. 1999. 'El movimiento higienista español ante el 98.' In *Los significados del 98: la sociedad española en la génesis del siglo XX*. Ed. Octavio Ruiz-Manjón Cabeza and María Alicia Langa Laorga, 393–402. Madrid: Fundación ICO, Biblioteca Nueva, Universidad Complutense de Madrid.

'Cárceles: Miedo al SIDA.' 1986. *El Dominical*. Madrid: RTVE.

Centers for Disease Control and Prevention. 1981. 'Pneumocystis Pneumonia – Los Angeles.' *Mortality and Morbidity Weekly Report* 30 (21): 250–52.

———. 1982a. 'A Cluster of Kaposi's Sarcoma and Pneumocystis Carinii Pneumonia among Homosexual Male Residents of Los Angeles and Range Counties, California.' *Mortality and Morbidity Weekly Report* 31 (23): 305–07.

———. 1982b. 'Pneumocystis Carinii Pneumonia among Persons with Hemophilia A.' *Mortality and Morbidity Weekly Report* 31 (27): 365–67.

———. 1984. 'Update: Acquired Immunodeficiency Syndrome (AIDS) in Persons with Hemophilia.' *Mortality and Morbidity Weekly Report* 33 (42): 589–91.

———. 1986. 'Update: Acquired Immunodeficiency Syndrome – Europe.' *Mortality and Morbidity Weekly Report* 35 (3): 35–38, 43–46.

——. 2015. 'Leading Causes of Death Reports, 1981–1998.' *Fatal Injury Queries* (blog). June 24, 2015. https://webappa.cdc.gov/sasweb/ncipc/leadcaus9.html.

Cohen, Ed. 2009. *A Body Worth Defending: Immunity, Biopolitics, and the Apotheosis of the Modern Body.* Durham, NC: Duke University Press.

Coordinadora de Frentes de Liberación Homosexual del Estado Español. 1982. *Ni represión / Ni discriminación / Tal como eres gana la calle.* Poster.

Córdoba, David, Javier Sáez, and Francisco Javier Vidarte, eds. 2005. *Teoría queer: políticas bolleras, maricas, trans, mestizas.* Barcelona: Egales.

Criado, Azucena. 1993. 'La Administración anuncia que indemnizará a los hemofílicos infectados con el virus del sida.' *El País*, March 10, 1993. http://elpais.com/diario/1993/03/10/sociedad/731718010_850215.html.

Crimp, Douglas. 2002. *Melancholia and Moralism: Essays on AIDS and Queer Politics.* Cambridge, MA: MIT Press.

D. 1983. 'Los vecinos de Arganzuela, hartos de robos y asaltos.' *ABC*, February 11, 1983.

Davis, Ryan. 2013. *The Spanish Flu: Narrative and Cultural Identity in Spain, 1918.* New York: Palgrave Macmillan.

De Lauretis, Teresa. 1991. 'Queer Theory: Lesbian and Gay Sexualities.' *Differences: A Journal of Feminist Cultural Studies* 3 (2): iii–xviii.

Diedrich, Lisa. 2016. *Indirect Action: Schizophrenia, Epilepsy, AIDS, and the Course of Health Activism.* Minneapolis: University of Minnesota Press.

Drescher, Jack. 2015. 'Queer Diagnoses Revisited: The Past and Future of Homosexuality and Gender Diagnoses in DSM and ICD.' *International Review of Psychiatry* 27 (5): 386–95.

Dubler, Nancy Neveloff, and Victor W. Sidel. 1991. 'AIDS and the Prison System.' In *A Disease of Society: Cultural and Institutional Responses to AIDS.* Ed. Dorothy Nelkin, David P. Willis, and Scott Parris, 71–83. New York: Cambridge University Press.

Dunn, Kate. 1993. 'HIV and Canada's Hemophiliacs: Looking Back at a Tragedy.' *Canadian Medical Association Journal* 148 (4): 609–12.

Edelman, Lee. 2004. *No Future: Queer Theory and the Death Drive.* Durham, NC: Duke University Press.

Edensor, Tim. 2005. 'The Ghosts of Industrial Ruins: Ordering and Disordering Memory in Excessive Space.' *Environment and Planning D: Society and Space* 23 (6): 829–49. https://doi.org/10.1068/d58j.

EHGAM. 1985. 'Día mundial de la liberación gay y lesbiana.' Flyer.

'EL SIDA.' 1985. *Generación 800.* Madrid: RTVE.

'El SIDA en San Francisco: Pánico en las calles.' 1985. *Informe Semanal.* Madrid: RTVE.

Epps, Brad. 2009. 'Retos, riesgos, pautas y promesas de la teoría queer.' *Revista Iberoamericana* 74 (225): 897–920. https://doi.org/10.5195/REVIBEROAMER.2008.5216.

Esposito, Roberto. 2011. *Immunitas: The Protection and Negation of Life.* Malden, MA: Polity.

Estruch, R., A. Urbano Ispizua, J. Pedro-Botet Montoya, C. Cuturi, A. Urbano-Márquez, and C. Rozman. 1983. 'Síndrome de inmunodeficiencia adquirida en un varón residente en Barcelona.' *Medicina Clínica* 81 (14): 645.

Federación Española de Hemofilia. 1993. 'Editorial.' *Fedhemo: Federación Española de Hemofília* 1 (1): 5.
Feinberg, Matthew I. 2022. *From the Theater to the Plaza: Spectacle, Protest, and Urban Space in Twenty-First-Century Madrid*. Montreal: McGill-Queen's University Press.
Feldman, Eric A, and Ronald Bayer, eds. 1999. *Blood Feuds: AIDS, Blood, and the Politics of Medical Disaster*. New York: Oxford University Press.
Fernández de Alba, Francisco. 2020. *Sex, Drugs, and Fashion in 1970s Madrid*. Toronto Iberic 50. Toronto: University of Toronto Press.
Fin de siglo 1987. Madrid: RTVE.
Flesler, Daniela. 2008. *The Return of the Moor: Spanish Responses to Contemporary Moroccan Immigration*. West Lafayette, IN: Purdue University Press.
Fluvià, Armand de. 1978a. 'El movimiento homosexual en el estado español.' In *El homosexual ante la sociedad enferma*. Ed. José Ramón Enríquez, 145–67. Barcelona: Tusquets.
———. 1978b. 'La represión legal.' In *El homosexual ante la sociedad enferma*. Ed. José Ramón Enríquez, 72–93. Barcelona: Tusquets.
Foucault, Michel. 2003. *Abnormal: Lectures at the Collège de France, 1974–1975*. New York: Picador.
Franco, Jesús. 1986. *SIDA: La peste del siglo XX*. Unpublished film script. Madrid. Biblioteca Nacional de Madrid.
Fraser, Benjamin. 2009. *Deaf History and Culture in Spain: A Reader of Primary Documents*. Washington, DC: Gallaudet University Press.
Fuentes Peris, Teresa. 2003. *Visions of Filth: Deviancy and Social Control in the Novels of Galdós*. Liverpool: Liverpool University Press.
Gais per la Salut. 1987. 'Estima com vulguis / Estimga segur.' Flyer.
Gamella, Juan F. 1997. 'Heroína en España, 1977–1996. Balance de una crisis de drogas.' *Claves de Razón Práctica* 72: 20–30.
García-Rodríguez, José Angel. 1984. 'SIDA, precursor de una nueva patología infecciosa? Discurso pronunciado en la solemne apertura del Curso Académico 1984–1985.' Salamanca: Universidad de Salamanca.
Garfield, Simon. 2011. 'The Rise and Fall of AZT.' *The Independent*, October 23, 2011. https://www.independent.co.uk/arts-entertainment/rise-and-fall-azt-it-was-drug-had-work-it-brought-hope-people-hiv-and-aids-and-millions-company-developed-it-it-had-work-there-was-nothing-else-many-who-used-azt-it-didn-t-2320491.html. Accessed October 3, 2022.
Garijo, Adolfo, dir. 1987. *Carabanchel: la otra orilla*. Tele Prisión. Madrid: Radio Televisión Madrid.
Gelabert Blanes, A. 1987. 'Cribado de anticuerpos antivirus de la inmunodeficiencia humana en donantes de sangre.' *Medicina Clínica* 89 (1): 14–16.
Goldstein, Diane E. 2004. *Once Upon a Virus: AIDS Legends and Vernacular Risk Perception*. Logan: Utah State University Press.
González, Álvaro. 2020. 'Tele Prisión, la cadena de TV que pusieron en marcha los presos de Carabanchel en los 80.' *Valenciaplaza.Com*, February 1, 2020. https://valenciaplaza.com/tele-prision-la-cadena-de-tv-que-pusieron-en-marcha-los-presos-de-carabanchel-en-los-80. Accessed October 3, 2022.
González-Ruibal, Alfredo, and Carmen Ortiz. 2015. 'The Prison of Carabanchel (Madrid, Spain): A Life Story.' In *War and Cultural Heritage: Biographies of Place*, 128–55. Cambridge: Cambridge University Press.

Gould, Deborah B. 2009. *Moving Politics: Emotion and ACT UP's Fight against AIDS*. Chicago: University of Chicago Press.

Guasch, Óscar. 1991. 'SIDA y homosexualidad en España: una década de epidemia.' *Jano: Medicina y Humanidades* 40 (942): 77–86.

Heredia Urzáiz, Iván. 2009. 'Control y exclusión social: la Ley de Vagos y Maleantes en el primer Franquismo.' In *Universo de micromundos: VI Congreso de Historia Local de Aragón*, 109–22. Zaragoza: Institución Fernando el Católico.

Herranz Durández, Luisa. 2016. 'Biblioteca y aulario de la UNED en las antiguas escuelas pías de San Fernando de Madrid: análisis y crítica de su intervención.' Working paper. Máster en conservación y restauración del patrimonio arquitectónico. http://oa.upm.es/48118/.

Hogan, Erin K. 2018. *The Two cines con niño: Genre and the Child Protagonist in over Fifty Years of Spanish Film (1955–2010)*. Edinburgh: Edinburgh University Press.

Honig, Bonnie. 2013. *Antigone Interrupted*. Cambridge: Cambridge University Press.

'Invertir.' n.d. In *Real Academia Española*, 2018 ed. http://dle.rae.es/?id=M3VWBGW. Accessed July 27, 2018.

Jagose, Annamarie. 1996. *Queer Theory: An Introduction*. New York: New York University Press.

Keller, Patricia, and Jonathan Snyder. 2011. 'Encounters with the Unsightly: Reading (AIDS) History, Photography, and the Obscene.' Ed. Maria Nilsson. *Hispanic Issues On Line Debates*, On Photography, History, and Memory in Spain, 3 (spring): 91–115. https://cla.umn.edu/hispanic-issues/debates/photography-history-and-memory-spain. Accessed December 7, 2022.

Kornetis, Kostis. 2014. '"Is There a Future in This Past?" Analyzing 15M's Intricate Relation to the *Transición*.' *Journal of Spanish Cultural Studies* 15 (1–2): 83–98. https://doi.org/10.1080/14636204.2014.938432.

La Vanguardia. 1987. 'Editorial: El sida en las cárceles.' *La Vanguardia*, April 24, 1987, sec. Editorial.

Labanyi, Jo. 2002. 'Resemanticising Feminine Surrender: Cross-Gender Identifications in the Writings of Spanish Female Fascist Activists.' In *Women's Narrative and Film in 20th Century Spain*. Ed. Ofelia Ferrán and Kathleen Glenn, 75–94. New York: Routledge.

Larson, Susan, ed. 2021. *Architecture and the Urban in Spanish Film*. Bristol: Intellect. https://doi.org/10.1386/9781789384895.

Lawlor, Clark. 2006. *Consumption and Literature: The Making of the Romantic Disease*. New York: Palgrave Macmillan.

Lázaro-Reboll, Antonio, and Ian Olney, eds. 2018. *The Films of Jess Franco*. Detroit, MI: Wayne State University Press.

Llamas, Ricardo. 1994. 'La reconstrucción del cuerpo homosexual en tiempos de SIDA.' *Revista Española de Investigaciones Sociológicas* 68: 141–71.

Llamas, Ricardo, and Fefa Vila. 1994. 'Spain: Passion for Life. Una historia del movimiento de lesbianas y gays en el estado español.' In *ConCiencia de un singular deseo: estudios lesbianos y gays en el estado español*. Ed. Xosé M Buxán, 189–224. Barcelona: Laertes.

López Romo, Raúl. 2008. *Del gueto a la calle: el movimiento gay y lesbiano en el País Vasco y Navarra, 1975–1983*. Donostia-San Sebastián: Tercera Prensa.

Lucas, Tim. 1993. 'Introduction.' In *Obsession: The Films of Jess Franco*. Ed. Lucas Balbo and Peter Blumenstock, 13–30. Berlin: Graf Haufen & Frank Trebbin.

Martín Hernández, Rut. 2009. 'El SIDA ante la opinión pública: el papel de la prensa y las compañas de prevención estatales en la representación social del SIDA en España.' *Studium: Revista de Humanidades* 15: 237–68.

Martín Villar, J. 1979. 'Comunicación presentada en el Congreso Anual de la Asociación Española de Hematología y Hemoterapia.' *Nueva Imagen* 0 (June): 17–19.

Mbembe, Achille. 2001. *On the Postcolony*. Oakland, CA: University of California Press.

McKay, Richard A. 2014. '"Patient Zero": The Absence of a Patient's View of the Early North American AIDS Epidemic.' *Bulletin of the History of Medicine* 88 (1): 161–94. https://doi.org/10.1353/bhm.2014.0005.

Mendoza García, Joaquín. 1983. 'Entrevista: La Administración sigue sin dar solución a nuestros problemas.' *Nueva Imagen* 10–11 (June): 3–5.

Meruane, Lina. 2014. *Viral Voyages: Tracing AIDS in Latin America*. Trans. Andrea Rosenberg. New York: Palgrave Macmillan.

Miguel, Jesús M. de, and David L. Kirp. 1992. 'Spain: An Epidemic of Denial.' In *AIDS in the Industrialized Democracies: Passions, Politics, and Policies*. Ed. David L. Kirp and Ronald Bayer, 168–84. New Brunswick, NJ: Rutgers University Press.

Monferrer Tomàs, Jordi M. 2003. 'La construcción de la protesta en el movimiento gay español: la Ley de Peligrosidad Social (1970) como factor precipitante de la acción colectiva.' *Reis: Revista Española de Investigaciones Sociológicas* 102 (June): 171–204. https://doi.org/10.2307/40184541.

Moran, Dominique. 2015. *Carceral Geography: Spaces and Practices of Incarceration*. Farnham: Ashgate.

Murray, Thomas H. 1991. 'The Poisoned Gift: AIDS and Blood.' In *A Disease of Society: Cultural and Institutional Responses to AIDS*. Ed. Dorothy Nelkin, David P. Willis, and Scott Parris, 216–40. New York: Cambridge University Press.

Nazario. 1987. 'Folla seguro, o El misterio de navón.' Flyer.

Nelkin, Dorothy. 1999. 'Cultural Perspectives on Blood.' In *Blood Feuds: AIDS, Blood, and the Politics of Medical Disaster*. Ed. Eric A Feldman and Ronald Bayer, 273–92. New York: Oxford University Press.

Ngai, Sianne. 2007. *Ugly Feelings*. Cambridge, MA: Harvard University Press.

Nichols, William J., and H. Rosi Song, eds. 2014. *Toward a Cultural Archive of La Movida: Back to the Future*. Madison, NJ: Fairleigh Dickinson University Press.

Nirenberg, David. 2015. *Communities of Violence: Persecution of Minorities in the Middle Ages*. Princeton, NJ: Princeton Univeristy Press.

Olmeda, Fernando. 2004. *El látigo y la pluma: homosexuales en la España de Franco*. Madrid: Oberon.

Ortiz García, Carmen, and Mario Martínez Zauner. 2016. 'La cárcel de Carabanchel: lugar de memoria y memorias del lugar.' *Scripta Nova: Revista Electrónica de Geografía y Ciencias Sociales* 18, 493 (02): 1–19. https://revistes.ub.edu/index.php/ScriptaNova/issue/view/1289. Accessed December 7, 2022.

Pavlović, Tatjana. 2003. *Despotic Bodies and Transgressive Bodies: Spanish Culture from Francisco Franco to Jesús Franco*. Albany, NY: State University of New York Press.

Pérez-Sánchez, Gema. 2007. *Queer Transitions in Contemporary Spanish Culture: From Franco to La Movida*. Albany, NY: State University of New York Press.

Petit, Jordi. 2003. *25 años más: una perspectiva sobre le pasado, presente y futuro del movimiento de gays, lesbianas, bisexuales y transexuales*. Barcelona: Icaria.

Prádanos, Luis I. 2018. *Postgrowth Imaginaries: New Ecologies and Counterhegemonic Culture in Post-2008 Spain*. Liverpool: Liverpool University Press. https://doi.org/10.2307/j.ctvt6rjgt.

Relaño, Alfredo. 1983. 'Confirmado oficialmente que dos hermanos murieron en Sevilla a causa del síndrome de inmunodeficiencia.' *El País*, May 5. http://elpais.com/diario/1983/05/05/sociedad/420933603_850215.html. Accessed October 3, 2022.

Remacha, Belén. 2019. '30 años de campañas para prevenir el VIH: así se empezó a informar sobre el virus y se ideó el "Póntelo, Pónselo."' *ElDiario.Es*, November 27. https://www.eldiario.es/sociedad/sida-noda_1_1231937.html. Accessed October 3, 2022.

Rivas, Javier. 1985. 'La historia de Rafael.' *El País*, September 6. http://elpais.com/diario/1985/09/07/sociedad/494892005_850215.html. Accessed October 3, 2022.

Romero Vallecillos, Manuel, Eugenia Oviedo-Joekes, Joan Carles Mach Cerdà, and Iñaki Markez Alonso. 2005. 'Programas de Jeringuillas.' *Addiciones* 17 (2): 257–75.

Rozenbaum, W., J.P. Coulaud, A.G. Saimot, D. Klatzmann, C. Mayaud, and M.F. Carette. 1982. 'Multiple Opportunistic Infection in a Male Homosexual in France.' *The Lancet* 319 (8271): 572–73. https://doi.org/10.1016/S0140-6736(82)92087-6.

Sánchez, Esther. 1985. 'Vecinos de embajadores expulsan a unos delincuentes de un refugio ruinoso.' *ABC*, June 25, 1985.

Sánchez Ocaña, Ramón, dir. 1985. 'El SIDA.' *Más vale prevenir*. Madrid: RTVE.

——, dir. 1987. 'El SIDA.' *Más vale prevenir*. Madrid: RTVE.

Servicio Madrileño de Salud. n.d. 'Una necesidad social.' *Donación de Sangre* (blog). http://www.madrid.org/cs/Satellite?cid=1259569861861&language=es&pagename=PortalSalud/Page/PTSA_pintarContenidoFinal&vest=1259499533482#. Accessed January 13, 2017.

Shilts, Randy. 1987. *And the Band Played On: Politics, People, and the AIDS Epidemic*. New York: St. Martin's Press.

'SIDA: Crece la alarma.' 1985. *El Dominical*. Madrid: RTVE.

'SIDA: La enfermedad de los 80.' 1983. *Informe Semanal*. Madrid: RTVE. http://www.rtve.es/alacarta/videos/informe-semanal/sida-enfermedad-80-informe-semanal-1983/1118964/. Accessed October 3, 2022.

SIDA STUDI. 2011. '30 años de VIH/SIDA, 30 años de luchas: 1° diciembre: día mundial de lucha contra el SIDA.' Barcelona: Sida Studi. http://www.sidastudi.org/es/registro/d25f080433caee870133d9af2b160013. Accessed October 3, 2022.

Smith, Paul Julian. 1996. *Vision Machines: Cinema, Literature, and Sexuality in Spain and Cuba, 1983–93*. London: Verso.

Sontag, Susan. 1990. *Illness as Metaphor and AIDS and its Metaphors*. New York: Doubleday.

Sosa-Velasco, Alfredo. 2010. *Médicos escritores en España, 1885–1955: Santiago Ramón y Cajal, Pío Baroja, Gregorio Marañón y Antonio Vallejo Nágera*. Colección Támesis. Serie A, Monografías 286. Woodbridge: Tamesis.

Stockton, Kathryn Bond. 2009. *The Queer Child, or Growing Sideways in the Twentieth Century*. Durham, NC: Duke University Press.

Thomas, Sarah. 2019. *Inhabiting the In-between: Childhood and Cinema in Spain's Long Transition*. Toronto: University of Toronto Press.

Treichler, Paula A. 1999. *How to Have Theory in an Epidemic: Cultural Chronicles of AIDS*. Durham, NC: Duke University Press.

Tusell, Joan M. 1993. 'Avances científicos y perspectivas de futuro en hemofília.' *Fedhemo: Federación Española de Hemofília* 1 (2): 13–18.

Usó, Juan Carlos. 1996. *Drogas y cultura de masas: España, 1855–1995*. Madrid: Taurus.

Vila Núñez, Fefa. 1999. 'Genealogías feministas: contribuciones de la perspectiva radical a los estudios de las mujeres.' *Política y Sociedad* 32: 43–51.

Vilaseca, J., J.M. Arnau, R. Bacardi, C. Mieras, A. Serrano, and C. Navarro. 1982. 'Kaposi's Sarcoma and Toxoplasma Gondii Brain Abscess in a Spanish Homosexual.' *The Lancet* 319 (8271): 572.

Villace, Dacio. 1982. 'La hemofilia explicada a los niños.' *Nueva Imagen* 8–9 (December): 6–8.

Wald, Priscilla. 2008. *Contagious: Cultures, Carriers, and the Outbreak Narrative*. Durham, NC: Duke University Press.

Wheeler, Duncan. 2020. *Following Franco: Spanish Culture and Politics in Transition, 1962–92*. Manchester: Manchester University Press.

Whittaker, Tom. 2020. *The Spanish Quinqui Film: Delinquency, Sound, Sensation*. Manchester: Manchester University Press.

Williams, Linda. 1991. 'Film Bodies: Gender, Genre, and Excess.' *Film Quarterly* 44 (4): 2–13. https://doi.org/10.2307/1212758.

Williams, Raymond. 2009. *Marxism and Literature*. Oxford: Oxford University Press.

Woodard, Vincent, Justin A. Joyce, and Dwight A. McBride. 2014. *The Delectable Negro: Human Consumption and Homoeroticism within U.S. Slave Culture*. New York: New York University Press.

World Health Organization. 2017. 'The Top 10 Causes of Death.' *Media Centre* (blog). January 2017. http://www.who.int/mediacentre/factsheets/fs310/en/.

——. 2018. 'ICD-11: Classifying Disease to Map the Way We Live and Die.' *International Classification of Diseases* (blog). June 18, 2018. https://www.who.int/health-topics/international-classification-of-diseases.

Wright, Sarah. 2013. *The Child in Spanish Cinema*. Manchester: Manchester University Press.

Index

Printed and bound by CPI Group (UK) Ltd, Croydon, CR0 4YY

13/09/2026

14961098-0004